TENS: Clinical Applications and Related Theory

Deirdre M. Walsh BPhysiotherapy DPhil MISCP MCSP
Lecturer in Physiotherapy, University of Ulster, Northern Ireland

With a contribution by
Eric T. McAdams BSc(Hons) Engineering DPhil MIEEE
Reader, School of Electrical and Mechanical Engineering,
University of Ulster, Northern Ireland

Foreword by
Norman Shealy MD PhD
Founder, Shealy Institute for Comprehensive Health Care Springfield, USA

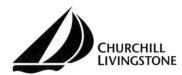 CHURCHILL
LIVINGSTONE

NEW YORK EDINBURGH LONDON MADRID MELBOURNE SAN FRANCISCO AND TOKYO 1997

18999875

CHURCHILL LIVINGSTONE
Medical Division of Pearson Professional Limited

Distributed in the United States of America by Churchill
Livingstone, 650 Avenue of the Americas, New York, N.Y.
10011, and by associated companies, branches and
representatives throughout the world.

© Pearson Professional Limited 1997

First published 1997

ISBN 0 443 05323 5

British Library Cataloguing in Publication Data
A catalogue record for this book is available from the British
Library.

Library of Congress Cataloging in Publication Data
A catalog record for this book is available from the Library
of Congress.

Note
Medical knowledge is constantly changing. As new
information becomes available, changes in treatment,
procedures, equipment and the use of drugs become
necessary. The editors/authors/contributors and the
publishers have, as far as it is possible, taken care to ensure
that the information given in this text is accurate and up-to-
date. However, readers are strongly advised to confirm that
the information, especially with regard to drug usage,

The
publisher's
policy is to use
paper manufactured
from sustainable forests

Printed in Singapore

Contents

Foreword   **vii**

Preface   **ix**

Acknowledgements   **xi**

Glossary   **xiii**

1. Introduction and historical perspective   **1**

2. Pain and its modulation   **11**

3. TENS: physiological principles and stimulation parameters   **25**

4. Basic electronic and electrode principles   **41**
   Eric McAdams

5. Review of experimental studies on TENS   **63**

6. Review of clinical studies on TENS   **83**

7. The clinical application of TENS   **103**

8. Non-analgesic effects of TENS   **125**

9. Interesting developments and the future of TENS   **139**

10. TENS systems   **143**

Appendix I   Transient responses and nonlinearity   **155**
Eric McAdams

Index   **161**

Foreword

Since at least 47 AD, when Scribonius Largus reported on the cure of the pain of gout by accidental contact with a torpedo fish, or electric ray, electrotherapy has captured the imagination of many therapists. In 1745, medical applications of electrotherapy moved closer to our modern concept with the use of the electrostatic generator. No less than John Wesley, founder of the Methodist Church, who also was a physician, commented favourably upon electrotherapy. It was towards the end of the 19th century that the precursors of TENS were developed. A wide variety of battery powered stimulators was marketed by Sears, Roebuck and Company, and other distributors. The sole survivor of this technology was the Electreat®, patented in 1919, and based upon earlier models. This particular model was sold at a rate of as many as 60 000 units per year, as late as the 1930s, but in 1941, the American FDA practically put them out of business by insisting that they could not advertise 'Electreat relieves pain'.

When I became interested in the possible use of electrotherapy in 1965, after reading Pat Wall and Ron Melzack's paper, 'The Gate Control of Pain' (Melzack & Wall 1965), I remembered the Electreat and literally begged engineers to make me a modern, solid-state Electreat device. It was almost a decade later that the first modern TENS devices were produced, first by Stimulation Technology, and within 2 weeks thereafter, by Medtronic, Inc. Unfortunately, no pharmaceutical company has ever promoted TENS in the USA and it has never caught on with the medical profession. It is certainly not as easy to use as a prescription pad, but it is infinitely more effective.

More importantly, none of the TENS has ever reproduced the output of the old Electreat. Only within the last few years, have we demonstrated the reason why this device is superior to all of the modern TENS. It includes frequencies up to 78 gigaherz, or billion cycles per second, which we have found to be considerably more effective than most other TENS devices. The electronics of the Electreat have now been reworked, adding voltage regulation and constant current output, and, interestingly, this device now allows the sensory perception of spreading of the current up to 12 inches (30.5 cm) above and below the electrodes, and is considerably more effective in relieving pain.

However, even the modern devices without the gigaherz frequencies are highly effective, most particularly in acute pain, where, 80% of the time, acute pain can be managed without the use of drugs when the TENS device is properly applied. In chronic pain, modern TENS devices are primarily effective only about 50% of the time. Nevertheless, they are better than any drug on the market and, except for the caveat that they should not be used in patients with cardiac pacemakers, there are virtually no complications in the use of TENS.

In recent months, we have demonstrated that the use of the Liss TENS, a very specific, moderately high, frequency device (15 000 cycles per second modulated at 15 and 500 Hz), when applied to 12 specific acupuncture points, both raises DHEA, or dehydroepi-androsterone, and provides striking relief in patients with migraine headache, both prophylactically and acutely.

We, at the Shealy Institute, are delighted that Dr Walsh has presented such a comprehensive approach in *TENS: Clinical Applications and Related Theory*. With its publication we hope that modern electrotherapy will take its appropriate place as the treatment of choice in acute pain, and in chronic pain, of virtually all causes. Dr Walsh's book is by far the most comprehensive and detailed that has been presented to date. We hope that every family physician, every emergency ward physician, every internist and surgeon and every physical therapist will read this important work and allow it to assist them in comprehensive management of pain.

N.S.

REFERENCE

Melzack R, Wall P D 1965 Pain mechanisms: a new theory. Science 150: 971–979

Preface

Although electricity has been effectively used in pain management for many centuries, transcutaneous electrical nerve stimulation (TENS) can be classed as a product of the early 1970s. In spite of wide availability for almost 3 decades, there is still considerable ambiguity regarding the clinical potential of this modality and indeed, its modus operandi. This is reflected in the response obtained from a recent questionnaire survey of chartered physiotherapists (see Ch. 1), who expressed dissatisfaction with the amount of available tests and published articles on TENS; only 18.8% of respondents felt satisfied with the amount of literature available to them. My own experiences as an undergraduate and postgraduate physiotherapist heightened my awareness of the confusion surrounding the selection of an optimal TENS treatment regime for pain relief.

The primary aim of this text is to try to answer many of the questions asked about TENS by three different groups: the student, the practising clinician and the researcher, or indeed any combination of the three. I have had the privilege of being interested in TENS from all three perspectives; therefore, in this text, I have tried to answer all the questions that I might have asked as a student, a practising physiotherapist and a research physiotherapist.

In writing this book, I felt it was important to take a comprehensive approach so that the reader could truly appreciate TENS at all levels. The information in the text is therefore delivered at three different levels – the essential background knowledge, the applied knowledge, and thirdly, the relevant research knowledge. I have endeavoured to do this in a concise fashion and, where possible, supported the text by examples and illustrations.

Finally, I sincerely hope that this text will better inform clinicians on all aspects of TENS so that they are then in a position to utilise it to its maximum potential for the relief of pain.

I would like to dedicate this book to my mother, who was the first person to teach me about TENS from her own personal experience.

D.M.W.

Acknowledgements

I would like to thank a number of people for their various and sometimes unknowing contributions to this book. To all my patients who have experienced any type of pain, your suffering gave me the ultimate reason to write this text; I humbly hope that this book will in some way contribute to a more effective conservative management of pain. To all my lecturers, undergraduate clinical supervisors and postgraduate supervisors, thank you most sincerely for answering my numerous questions which ultimately served to enhance my dual role as researcher and clinician. A special thanks to Mrs Claire O'Donnell, UCD School of Physiotherapy, who first encouraged me to pursue a career in research. Professor David Baxter, University of Ulster, who did such a good job in convincing me that I did want to write a book, thanks for being a pillar of support and for providing the much appreciated motivation during the various stages of writing, especially in the final stages. My colleagues from the University of Ulster, Dr Andrea Lowe, Mr Panos Barlas and Mr Tony Feenan, very kindly gave their time to produce several photographs for the text. A special thanks also to the library staff at the University who broke world records in returning research papers to me at the most crucial time. Mr Keith Tippey, Nidd Valley Medical Ltd, kindly clarified many questions on technical and legislative matters. My family, who have always provided unconditional support for my career, thanks for always being there for me. To my many friends in Belfast and Dublin from the clinical world, the academic world and the social world, thank you for your patience and understanding. A special thanks to Dr Pauline Wedlock who continually gave such positive support, especially towards the end. The help and support of the staff at Churchill Livingstone was also much appreciated. Finally, last but by no means least, I would like to thank Stephen for his love, understanding and patience, without which this book would never have been completed.

Glossary

AAMI	Association for the Advancement of Medical Instrumentation		ITEPI	instantaneous trailing edge pulse impedance
AC	alternating current		LBP	low back pain
ANOVA	analysis of variance		LCD	liquid-crystal display
ASIS	anterior superior iliac spine		LST	lateral spinothalamic tract
ATP	adenosine triphosphate			
			MAS	multisynaptic ascending system
BP	blood pressure		MPQ	McGill Pain Questionnaire
BSI	British Standards Institution		MPT	mechanical pain threshold
CABG	coronary artery bypass graft		NE	noradrenergic
CAP	compound action potential		NMES	neuromuscular electrical stimulation
CBM	cognitive behaviour modification		NRM	nucleus raphe magnus
CFPT	C fibre pain threshold		NS	nociceptive specific
CNS	central nervous system		NSAI	National Standards Authority of Ireland
CGRP	calcitonin gene related peptide			
CSF	cerebrospinal fluid		NSAID	non-steroidal anti-inflammatory drug
			NWC	number of words chosen
DC	direct current			
DCS	dorsal column stimulation		OA	osteoarthritis
DOMS	delayed onset muscle soreness			
DPSS	descending pain suppression system		PAG	periaqueductal grey matter
			PCA	patient controlled analgesia
ECG	electrocardiography		PEFR	peak expiratory flow rate
EFTA	European Free Trade Association		PEME	pulsed electromagnetic energy
EMG	electromyography		PNF	proprioceptive neuromuscular facilitation
ENS	electrical nerve stimulation			
			PPI	present pain intensity
FES	functional electrical stimulation		PRI	pain rating index
FEV	forced expiratory volume			
FVC	forced vital capacity		RA	rheumatoid arthritis
			RCT	randomised controlled trial
IASP	International Association for the Study of Pain		RF	reticular formation

ROM	range of movement		TENS	transcutaneous electrical nerve stimulation
RVM	rostral ventral medulla		TES	transcutaneous electrical stimulation
SD	strength–duration		TNS	transcutaneous nerve stimulation
SEP	somatosensory evoked potential			
SETT	submaximal effort tourniquet technique		UV	ultraviolet
SG	substantia gelatinosa		VAS	visual analogue scale
SPA	stimulation produced analgesia		VIP	vasoactive intestinal polypeptides
STT	spinothalamic tract			
			WDR	wide dynamic range
TCM	traditional Chinese medicine			

CHAPTER CONTENTS

Introduction and the need for the current text   1
Historical perspective   2
Terminology   4
TENS units and electrodes   4
Advantages of TENS   5
Disadvantages of/adverse reactions to TENS   5
Uses of TENS   5
   Electroacupuncture   7
Current standards and availability of TENS units   7

Summary of key points   8

1

Introduction and historical perspective

INTRODUCTION AND THE NEED FOR THE CURRENT TEXT

Transcutaneous electrical nerve stimulation (TENS) is the application of electrical stimulation to the skin via surface electrodes to stimulate nerve fibres, primarily for pain relief. Although the role of electricity in pain management has been acknowledged for many centuries, most progress in the use of electroanalgesia has been made in the past 30 years, following an improved understanding of pain mechanisms and the development of small, portable, battery-operated devices. Since the mid 1960s, our knowledge of the neuropharmacology and neurophysiology of pain has expanded considerably with the discovery and isolation of opioids and the publication of the gate control theory of pain. A subsequent period of prolific activity in research and clinical studies on electrical stimulation for pain relief became somewhat dormant within a few years. However, it has been encouraging to note that, since 1990, there has been an increase in the number of published papers on both clinical and experimental studies conducted in this area.

Although TENS units, as we know them today, have been available since the early 1970s, there is still a need for a better understanding and knowledge of the mechanisms of action of this modality and its diverse potential in pain management. Despite wide availability and popularity in the clinical field, there is still a deficiency in awareness of the optimal treatment parameters of TENS. The majority of physiotherapy depart-

1

ments and private practice clinics have at least one TENS unit, but quite often its potential is not realised, due, perhaps, to a degree of scepticism combined with a lack of neurophysiological knowledge, and also to the scarcity of available comprehensive texts.

In a recent survey of chartered physiotherapists (n = 639), a remarkably high number of clinicians (81.2%) were dissatisfied with the amount of information on TENS available to them (D M Walsh et al, unpublished work, 1995); the author has received similar feedback from clinicians attending study days and departmental seminars. It has become apparent over the past few years that there is a need for a text which can provide the essential information for the student, for the practising clinician and for the researcher. Thus, in writing the current text, this target audience was always kept in mind.

This first chapter introduces the reader to TENS by providing a historical account of the use of electricity for pain relief since the Egyptian era. A brief introduction to TENS follows, highlighting its advantages and disadvantages; the current uses of TENS are outlined and two recent surveys among chartered physiotherapists are used to highlight current applications of TENS and its popularity. Finally, comparisons are made between the availability of TENS units and between manufacturers' standards in Europe and the USA.

Historical perspective

The first use of electricity as a therapeutic modality did not involve a portable stimulator with an array of diodes and resistors but, rather, certain species of fish which contained organs that produce an electric charge, such as *Torpedo mamorata*, *Malapterurus electricus* and *Gymnotus electricus*. Typically, the fish was placed in contact with the area of the body experiencing pain to produce a series of electric shocks. Indeed, as far back as ancient Egypt, stone carvings in tombs from the Fifth Dynasty (about 2500 BC) depict the use of *Malapterurus electricus* (a species of catfish found in the River Nile) for the treatment of painful conditions. So, even at this early stage

our ancestors had realised the potential of electricity in the management of pain. Scribonius Largus (AD 46), one of the first Roman physicians, is believed to be the author of the earliest documentation on electrotherapy; in his work *Compositiones Medicae* he advocated the following treatment for gout:

For any type of gout a live black torpedo should, when the pain begins, be placed under the feet. The patient must stand on a moist shore washed by the sea and he should stay like this until his whole foot and leg up to the knee is numb. This takes away present pain and prevents pain from coming on if it has not already arisen. . .   (Kellaway 1946)

It is interesting to note that the depiction of electric fish in Egyptian tomb reliefs antedates the first written description of electrotherapy by several thousand years.

This crude methodology of electrical stimulation, as developed by the ancients, did not really improve until the 1700s, with the introduction of the Leyden jar in 1745. A major milestone, this device could both generate and store quantities of electric charge, thereby providing a pre-battery power source for electrical stimulation analgesia. During the 1800s, the development of the battery and the induction coil added further sophistication to electrotherapy. With such improvements in technology, electrotherapy supporters embarked upon a period of enthusiastic clinical activity; one of these supporters was John Wesley, founder of Methodism. In 1759, he published an early text detailing electrotherapy applications entitled *The Desideratum: or Electricity Made Plain and Useful*. The following is an example of a typical case history taken from this text:

Elenor Story, living in Clerkenwell Churchyard, catching cold, was seized with pain and weakness in the small of her back, as if it had been broke. By following the prescriptions of Dr. L., the pain after a fortnight settled in her shoulder. There it continued so violent, that often she had scarce any use of her arm. She afterward used abundance of remedies for above two years, but all to no effect. On Tuesday March 24, 1757, she received two strong shocks on each shoulder, which made the skin red and sore. That night she was in more pain than usual, trembled all over, and could get little sleep. The next morning she received several shocks all over, and so on Thursday morning and evening. After the second time her pain was gone, and she had the full use of both her arms.

(Wesley 1759)

The introduction of electroanalgesia into the medical profession was met with a considerable degree of scepticism; the inevitable opposition to this new concept, combined with variable clinical results, led to a decline in interest towards the end of the 19th century. This lack of interest continued until the 1960s, when the publication of the gate control theory and the introduction of dorsal column stimulation (DCS) rekindled interest in electrotherapy. The gate control theory, published by Melzack & Wall in 1965, provided a neurophysiological substrate for electrical stimulation analgesia which subsequently acted as a catalyst to the commercial production of electrical stimulators. Basically, this theory proposed that a 'gate' existed in the dorsal horn of the spinal cord which could control the volume of incoming nociceptive traffic (see Ch. 2 for more detail). Wall & Sweet (1967) provided clinical evidence to support this theory when they reported the success of high frequency *percutaneous* electrical nerve stimulation for the relief of chronic neurogenic pain.

Figure 1.1 illustrates the Electreat® apparatus, one of the first TENS-like devices, which was available in the USA as far back as 1919. This apparatus was subsequently regarded as the original TENS device because it was the only electrical stimulation device for pain control

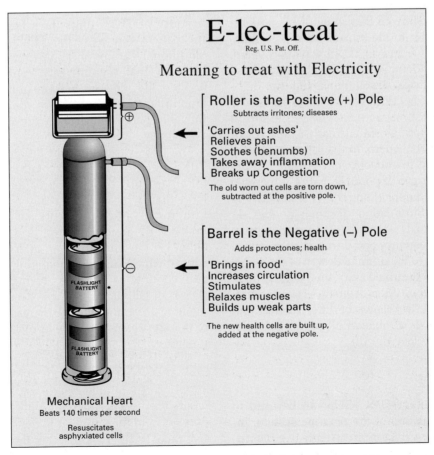

Figure 1.1 The Electreat was a very early electrical stimulation apparatus which was available for purchase in the USA as early as 1919 (courtesy of Dr Norman Shealy, Shealy Institute, Missouri, USA).

which was still being manufactured in the USA at the time the gate control theory was published (Long 1991).

The second contributing factor for renewed interest in electrical stimulation around this time was the development of dorsal column stimulation (DCS), a new technique for pain relief. DCS involves surgical implantation of electrodes in the dorsal column of the spinal cord which are activated by an external battery-operated device (Shealy et al 1967). Dr Norman Shealy initially used the battery-operated Electreat stimulator as a screening device to establish patients' candidacy for DCS (Shealy 1974): if the patients responded favourably to a trial of such external transcutaneous stimulation, this was taken as an indication that they would respond positively to DCS. Interestingly, preliminary results from Shealy's work showed that some of his patients responded better to the transcutaneous stimulation than to DCS and so TENS was discovered, almost by accident. This discovery initiated a new era of electrical stimulation analgesia.

Meyer & Fields (1972) were among the first to report the clinical use of *transcutaneous* electrical nerve stimulation (as we currently know it) for the relief of chronic pain. In the following years, researchers and manufacturers combined to develop several types of portable, battery-operated electrical stimulators (Long 1974, Shealy 1974), such as the Stimulation Technology EPC-1® model (Stimtech, USA) which allowed manipulation of pulse frequency and duration parameters. Improvements to the original design of the TENS apparatus has continued since then so that there is currently a multitude of manufacturers offering a variety of stimulators of different sizes and shapes as well as a range of adjustable stimulation parameters (see Ch. 10).

Terminology

Technically, the acronym TENS can be used to cover all stimulators of the nervous system, including muscle stimulation currents, e.g. neuromuscular electrical stimulation (NMES) and functional electrical stimulation (FES); typically, however, TENS is used solely to refer to those devices used for pain relief. Alternative acronyms used to describe these devices are TNS (transcutaneous nerve stimulation) and TES (transcutaneous electrical stimulation). In terms of electrotherapy classification, TENS is classed as a low frequency current.

TENS units and electrodes

A variety of TENS models are currently available ranging from single or dual channel to multichannel units. The single and dual channel units are invariably operated by a 9 V battery whereas multichannel units tend to be powered by mains electricity. The design of the TENS unit has now reached the advanced stage that the smallest unit currently available is only 5.5 cm in length and 6 g in weight (Unitouch®, Tenscare, UK). The majority of TENS units have belt clips so that the patient can wear the TENS while mobile. Additional features on TENS units include safety locks so that the intensity control cannot be accidentally adjusted. In some units all the stimulation parameter controls are concealed by a removable panel which also prevents accidental adjustment.

The wide variety of unit design means that a TENS device can now be tailored specifically for a particular patient population (for example, large dials which can be easily manipulated are ideal for an arthritic patient). An obstetric TENS unit has the unique feature of a trigger switch either on the unit or on an attached hand-held control which facilitates changing between burst and continuous outputs during the different phases of labour. All of these designs have been made to accommodate the increasing popularity of this device and its wide application in clinical medicine.

There is an even broader range of types and sizes of electrodes used with TENS. The original TENS electrode was made of carbon rubber which was covered evenly with conductive gel (wet gel) and then applied to the skin with adhesive tape. In the past 10 years the production of the disposable hydrogel pad has made the application of TENS even more user-friendly; the hydrogel pad is applied directly to the carbon rubber electrode instead of the wet gel typically employed, which cuts down on the 'mess' associated with the application of the latter. Probably the most popular choice of electrode is the self-adhesive type which comes in a variety of shapes and sizes which can effectively mould to irregularly shaped areas of the body. This type of electrode has the advantage that it is very easy for both the clinician and patient to apply; however, it is more expensive.

Advantages of TENS

There are a number of advantages of TENS which make it appealing to both the clinician and the patient:

- TENS is a non-invasive device.
- It is portable.
- TENS is user-friendly and safe to be used by the patient at home. It therefore offers the patient a self-management option – a desirable aspect of any treatment programme since this has been shown to increase patient compliance and response to treatment.
- After the initial cost of purchasing a TENS device, the replacement of batteries and electrodes are the main running costs. In long-standing cases of pain, this is cheaper than regular prescriptions for analgesics.
- The precautions and contraindications associated with TENS are few and are largely based on common sense. In addition, side-effects are minimal (i.e. skin irritation).
- TENS is non-addictive.

Disadvantages of/adverse reactions to TENS

Compared with the advantages listed above, the disadvantages of TENS are minimal. A number of patients cannot tolerate the sensation of electrical stimulation and invariably will not respond to a TENS treatment programme. Adverse responses to TENS are rare: mainly skin irritation due to allergic reaction to the conductive medium or tape. In many cases this can be remedied (if the source of irritation is known) by the substitution of an alternative medium or product.

As with any therapeutic electrical current, the danger of a thermal burn applies; this may occur due to a variety of reasons, e.g. if a very high current density should occur beneath the electrode. It should also be noted that the risk of a chemical burn is minimal as most TENS waveforms have a zero net DC component (see Ch. 3).

Uses of TENS

The development of solid-state electronics and subsequent production of small portable devices, as previously discussed, has greatly enhanced the application of electrical currents for the treatment of pain. As a result, TENS continues to gain popularity as an effective non-pharmacological modality in the management of pain. TENS is used as a pain-relieving modality by a range of clinicians including physiotherapists, general practitioners, podiatrists, nurses, dentists, chiropractors and acupuncturists. This notwithstanding, the most important user of TENS is the patient himself; this inherent advantage makes this modality unique compared to other electrotherapeutic modalities, e.g. ultrasound, low-intensity laser irradiation, etc.

It is imperative that the first point of contact for the pain patient who is considering TENS treatment is a properly trained clinician, who should make the appropriate steps to get a diagnosis for the pain if this is not already available. Beyond this, the input of a trained clinician is important not only for the precautions associated with TENS but also to establish an optimal treatment regime. The clinician has to choose from a range of stimulation parameters – frequency, pulse duration, output type and an additional range of electrode placement sites, e.g. over the painful area, spinal nerve roots, myotomes, etc.

The range of clinical applications of TENS in pain management includes low back pain, musculoskeletal pain, arthritic pain, obstetric pain and postoperative pain. While TENS is primarily and most widely used for pain relief, several non-analgesic effects of TENS have also been reported; these include promotion of wound healing, effects on the autonomic nervous system and antiemetic effects (discussed in greater detail in

Ch. 8). With these widespread applications and the advantages mentioned above, it is unfortunate that TENS is not more widely used in the management of pain. The popularity of TENS, along with the ambiguity surrounding its clinical application, is highlighted by the results of two recent surveys on the use of TENS. The first survey, by chartered physiotherapists in Northern Ireland, was carried out between 1993 and 1994 (D M Walsh et al, unpublished work, 1995). 639 chartered physiotherapists in Northern Ireland received a postal questionnaire requesting details of their use of TENS; a total of 181 completed questionnaires were returned. The survey included questions on:

- the type and source of instruction on TENS
- how TENS was rated for a range of painful conditions compared to other electrotherapeutic modalities
- what type of electrodes were used
- how stimulation parameters were chosen.

When asked about the source of their formal training on TENS, 42% of physiotherapists reported that it was from pre-registration training, 28.7% received instruction from within their department; other sources of formal training included lectures/study days (13.3%) and manufacturers' seminars (11.6%). The majority of informal training on TENS came from other staff within the department (66.8%), followed by information from books and journals (55.2%); however, a surprisingly high percentage (45.9%) of physiotherapists said that they used suppliers' literature for informal training. This reliance on manufacturers' literature needs to be addressed, not least because the treatment regimes recommended are seldom adequately supported by reference to published work.

The scarcity of comprehensive texts on TENS offers an explanation for the relatively low percentage of clinicians who reported that they got information from books and journals. Consequently, it was hardly surprising that only 18.8% of respondents felt satisfied by the amount of information available to them on TENS. The three most cited reasons for this dissatisfaction were as follows:

- lack of stimulation guidelines (79.1%)
- lack of formal instruction (66.2%)
- lack of published articles/books (33.1%).

Physiotherapists were also asked to rank TENS against a number of electrotherapeutic modalities (e.g. interferential therapy, laser, ultrasound) for six different painful conditions. TENS was ranked first for obstetric pain by 85.5% of respondents, and almost half of the respondents (47.3%) ranked it first for postoperative pain. In contrast, and perhaps surprisingly, interferential therapy ranked first for neurogenic pain, acute musculoskeletal pain and chronic musculoskeletal pain. Overall, interferential therapy appeared to be the most popular of the listed electrotherapeutic modalities and this became more apparent in a separate question where it was ranked first for both acute (44.1%) and chronic pain (44.8%) compared to the other modalities. In comparison, there was a considerable difference in physiotherapists' perceived effectiveness of TENS for acute pain (5.3%) compared to chronic pain (24.3%). This is something which might stem from a widespread myth that TENS should only be used for chronic pain. There is no reason why TENS should not be used for acute pain and, indeed, the high ranking of TENS for postoperative pain reflects this. Again, a lack of published literature in this area may be part of the reason for clinicians' apparent reluctance to use TENS for acute pain.

A more recent survey on the use and ownership of electrotherapeutic modalities in England has been carried out by Pope et al (1995). A total of 139 hospitals received a questionnaire and a high response rate was reported (83.5%). As more than one reply was received from several hospitals who had a number of specialist areas using electrotherapy, the total number of responses received was 213. The five most widely owned and used electrotherapeutic modalities were reported as being:

- ultrasound (n = 212)
- TENS (n = 201)
- interferential therapy applied via electrodes as opposed to suction electrodes (n = 196)

- pulsed shortwave diathermy (n = 190)
- flowtron (n = 188).

It was interesting to note that ownership/use of TENS units was very much on a par with interferential machines, yet in the Northern Ireland survey previously discussed, interferential therapy scored much higher than TENS for perceived effectiveness in a range of painful conditions. In Pope et al's survey (1995), a breakdown of the respondents on TENS showed that:

- 201 respondents owned and used TENS
- three respondents owned TENS but did not use it
- eight said they would like to purchase TENS
- only one respondent said they would not like to purchase TENS.

These two recent surveys undoubtedly highlight the popularity of TENS units, at least in the UK.

Electroacupuncture

In addition to the application of different modes of TENS (see Ch. 7), a TENS unit may also be used for electroacupuncture treatments. Electroacupuncture involves the application of an electrical current with parameters similar to acupuncture-like TENS (low frequency, high intensity and long pulse duration) to acupoints via needle or surface electrodes. Irrespective of whether the technique is invasive (needle electrode) or non-invasive (surface electrode), both types of electrode are connected to an electrical stimulator. Some electroacupuncture devices have a dual function in that they can locate acupuncture points as well as administering an electrical current. Acupuncture points typically have lower skin resistance (impedance) than the surrounding area and can therefore be located by applying a probe along the skin which measures skin resistance; when an area of decreased skin resistance is located, this is indicated by an audio or visual signal from the electroacupuncture unit which can then be switched to deliver an electrical current (and thus treatment) to the identified point.

Current standards and availability of TENS units

In the UK and Ireland, TENS units are typically prescribed by a clinician (most commonly a physiotherapist or GP). The majority of manufacturers will provide units on a trial basis or operate a rental system, particularly for obstetric TENS units when TENS is only used for a specified time period. In common with other medical devices, there are certain standards with which manufacturers have to comply before a TENS unit can be marketed. There are essentially two directives with which manufacturers have to comply within the European Community: the Medical Devices Directive and the Electromagnetic Compatibility Directive.

The Medical Devices Directive (93/42/EEC), which came into effect on 1 January 1995, is one of several directives regulating the safety and marketing of medical devices throughout the European Community. This means that any medical device which comes under this directive will have to comply with a set of standards which are common to all member states in the European Community. In addition, the European Free Trade Association (EFTA) member states have also agreed to implement these directives. The introduction of this directive means that medical devices sold in any member state will have reached a common standard and that there will be no inter-state trade barriers in the European Community.

There is a transitional period for the Medical Devices Directive (until 13 June 1998); during this transitional period, manufacturers will have the choice of either following existing national controls (in the UK, for example, this refers to the standards laid down by the British Standards Institution, i.e. BS 5724 Part 1) or meeting the requirements of the directive. From 14 June 1998, all devices covered by this directive must carry 'CE marking' either on the device itself or on its packaging. This CE marking 'means that the device satisfies the requirements essential for it to be fit for its intended purpose' (Medical Devices Agency Directives Bulletin No. 8 1994). Each member state will have a competent authority which will carry out the requirements of the directive. In the UK, the competent authority is the Secretary of State for Health acting through the Medical Devices Directorate and in Ireland it is the National Standards Authority of Ireland (NSAI).

The second directive, the Electromagnetic Compatibility Directive (89/336/EEC) came into effect in Europe on 1 January 1992, with a transitional period until 31 December 1995. This directive requires manufacturers to minimise the risk associated with all electrical and electronic apparatus regarding electromagnetic disturbance. Since 1 January 1996, devices must have a CE marking to indicate that they comply with this directive.

Some UK and Irish manufacturers sell TENS units directly to the patient with the recommendation that TENS should only be used on a properly diagnosed pain condition. Over the past few years, it has become apparent that a few manufacturers have resorted to advertisements in the popular press with invitations for members of the general public to request a unit on trial. While this is obviously a potentially lucrative method of sales, it also carries with it the assumption that a patient does not necessarily have to be assessed, diagnosed or given operation instructions from a trained clinician. The author has witnessed at least one case in which a patient suffered severe skin irritation after using TENS for long periods with a totally inappropriate electrode application technique; in this case the only information the patient had was the inadequate literature supplied by the manufacturer.

The legislation regarding the sale of TENS units in the USA is tighter than European legislation in that units can only be purchased if prescribed by a clinician. The Association for the Advancement of Medical Instrumentation (AAMI) has published a document entitled *American National Standard for Transcutaneous Electrical Nerve Stimulators* (Association for the Advancement of Medical Instrumentation 1986) which details recommended standards for the use of TENS for pain relief. The document was developed by the TENS subcommittee of the AAMI neurosurgery committee, which comprises physicians, researchers and members of industry. The areas covered by this document include labelling requirements, device markings, patient and clinician information, safety and performance requirements and test procedures. Before bringing a new TENS model onto the market in the USA, a 510(k) application must be made to the Food and Drug Administration. If this application is successful, this permits the marketing of a new device which is equivalent to devices already marketed; this means that any new TENS model must have a 510(k) before it can be marketed.

SUMMARY OF KEY POINTS

1. TENS is an acronym for transcutaneous electrical nerve stimulation.

2. Electricity has been used for pain relief since the time of ancient Egypt; modern TENS units, however, were not developed until the 1970s.

3. TENS was used initially as a screening method for dorsal column stimulation.

4. Two recent surveys have indicated that although TENS is a popular electrotherapeutic modality, there is dissatisfaction among physiotherapists regarding the amount of literature/texts available which describe its application.

5. TENS manufacturers are obliged to comply with certain standards regarding safety, technical specifications, and interference with other apparatus.

REFERENCES

Association for the Advancement of Medical Instrumentation 1986 American National Standard for transcutaneous electrical nerve stimulators. ANSI/AAMI NS4, Arlington, VA

Kellaway P 1946 The William Osler Medal Essay. The part played by electric fish in the early history of bioelectricity and electrotherapy. Bulletin of the History of Medicine 20: 112–137

Long D M 1974 External electrical stimulation as a treatment of chronic pain. Minnesota Medicine 57: 195–198

Long D M 1991 Fifteen years of transcutaneous electrical stimulation for pain control. Stereotactic and Functional Neurosurgery 56: 2–19

Melzack R, Wall P D 1965 Pain mechanisms: a new theory. Science 150: 971–979

Meyer G A, Fields H L 1972 Causalgia treated by selective large fibre stimulation of peripheral nerve. Brain 95: 163–168

Pope G D, Mockett S P, Wright J P 1995 A survey of electrotherapeutic modalities: ownership and use in the NHS in England. Physiotherapy 81: 82–91

Shealy C N 1974 Six years' experience with electrical stimulation for control of pain. Advances in Neurology 4: 775–782

Shealy C N, Mortimer J T, Reswick J B 1967 Electrical inhibition of pain by stimulation of the dorsal column: preliminary clinical report. Anaesthesia and Analgesia 46: 489–491

Wall P D, Sweet W H 1967 Temporary abolition of pain in man. Science 155: 108–109

Wesley J 1759 The desideratum: or electricity made plain and useful by a lover of mankind and of common sense. Baillière, Tindall and Cox, London

CHAPTER CONTENTS

Introduction   11

Neurophysiology of pain   11
Acute and chronic pain   12
Nociceptors   13
Sensitisation   13
Activation of nociceptors   13
Initiation of an action potential   13
Afferent fibres   13
Nerve fibre classification system   14
Myelinated and unmyelinated fibres   14
First and second pain   14
Dorsal horn   14
Spinal tracts/pathways   15
Lateral spinothalamic tract   15
Multisynaptic ascending system   15
Brainstem structures   15
Thalamus   16
Cerebral cortex   16

Neuromodulation of pain   16
Peripheral level   17
Spinal segmental level   17
Supraspinal level   18
Cortical level   18

**Mechanisms of neuromodulation relevant to
TENS   18**
Physiological blocking effect   18
Segmental inhibition/gate control theory   18
Counterirritation   19
Placebo effect   19
Descending pain suppression system   20
Summary   21

The psychology of pain – an overview   22

Summary of key points   22

2

Pain and its modulation

INTRODUCTION

In order to understand how TENS, or any pain-relieving modality, achieves its effects, it is necessary to have a basic understanding of the nociceptive pathways. This does not imply an expert knowledge of neuroanatomy, but rather an appreciation of the relevant neural structures which are involved in the perception and modulation of pain. To this end, this chapter is divided into two main sections: the first section describes the neural pathways subserving pain and the second section describes the mechanisms underlying the neuromodulation of pain. This background knowledge, which is presented succinctly and with minimal complexity, will be required in later chapters with regard to the clinical application of TENS. Finally, an overview of the psychology of pain is provided.

NEUROPHYSIOLOGY OF PAIN

The experience of pain results from a physiological response to a noxious stimulus; it is subject to a wide range of influences and therefore there is considerable variation in the perception of pain between individuals. These influences include cultural differences, states of emotion and past experiences (Fig. 2.1).

Some authors use the terms 'pain' and 'nociception' interchangeably, a confusing mistake which can be avoided by appropriate definitions. The subcommittee on taxonomy of the International Association for the Study of Pain (IASP;

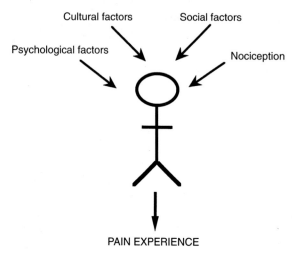

Figure 2.1 Factors which influence the pain experience.

Merskey et al 1979) has defined pain as 'a sensory and emotional experience associated with actual or potential tissue damage, or described in terms of such damage'. Pain should not be viewed exclusively as either a sensation or an emotion, since either assumption precludes particular characteristics necessary to the painful experience. Factors such as memory of previous experiences, psychological influences and pain tolerance variation cannot be accounted for by an isolated definition.

Additionally, it is incorrect to think that there is one rigid pathway which is responsible for the perception of pain; rather a multidimensional anatomical and physiological system is involved which takes a number of subjective factors into account. Physiologists tend to use the term 'nociception' to describe the specific response to a noxious stimulus, i.e. the transmission of noxious signals from the periphery to the cortex.

Acute and chronic pain

Pain can be described as acute or chronic: some texts provide definitions according to the temporal characteristics of each. However, it may be more appropriate to define acute and chronic pain in terms of the relationship between the symptoms and the underlying pathology. With acute pain, the body is responding to a noxious

stimulus which has caused damage, therefore the body's protective mechanism is activated and the symptoms reflect the underlying pathology. With chronic pain, typically the original pathology is healed so the symptom–pathology relationship is not as straightforward as before. In addition, due to the extra ramifications of chronic pain, the psychological aspects of pain must also be considered; these will be discussed at the end of the chapter.

In this first section, the chain of events which result in the perception of pain at a cortical level is outlined. Figure 2.2 summarises the anatomical pathways which are responsible for nociception; the components of these ascending nociceptive pathways, as we shall now call them, will be discussed separately in the following subsections.

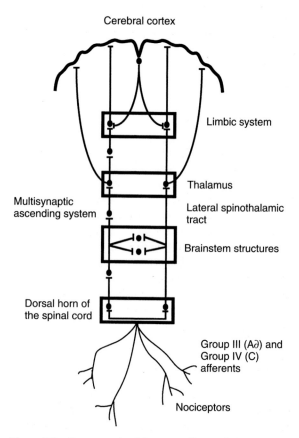

Figure 2.2 Components of the ascending nociceptive pathways.

Nociceptors

Noxious stimuli are no different from other stimuli in that they require a transducer to convert the appropriate stimulus, first into a receptor potential and subsequently into an action potential. Sensory receptors are specialised structures that respond selectively to specific stimuli and thus fulfil the role of transducers.

The receptor which responds to noxious stimuli is termed a nociceptor (*nocere* is the Latin for 'to injure'). Depending on the type of noxious stimuli to which they respond, nociceptors can be classified as:

- mechanical
- thermal
- polymodal.

Their structure is that of bare or free nerve endings and they are therefore the terminations of A∂ and C afferent fibres (see section on afferent fibres below). Nociceptors are found in nearly every type of tissue in the body and, compared with other receptors, they have a higher threshold for activation.

Sensitisation

One particular receptor property which is peculiar to nociceptors is sensitisation. This is the opposite of adaptation, a property which most of the other sensory receptors possess. Sensitisation means that if a noxious stimulus is maintained over a period of time, the threshold for activation of the nociceptor will be lowered and it therefore fires more rapidly. This is an important property which ensures that as long as a tissue damaging stimulus is present, the body is continuously kept aware of it and can therefore initiate the necessary protective response.

Activation of nociceptors

The activation of nociceptors is believed to occur through the release of certain chemical substances from the damaged tissue or the nerve terminals themselves (e.g., bradykinin, substance P, prostaglandins, serotonin).

Bradykinin. Bradykinin is a polypeptide which is formed in blood plasma in response to tissue damage.

Substance P. Substance P is another well recognised polypeptide which is found throughout the central and peripheral nervous system, including Group III and IV fibres, as well as non-neural elements. Several types of studies have indicated that substance P is a neurotransmitter involved in the transmission of nociceptive messages. The majority of this polypeptide, which is synthesised in cell bodies in dorsal root ganglia, is transported peripherally in the afferent neurone.

Prostaglandins. Prostaglandins are lipids which are synthesised in response to tissue damage from a variety of irritants – chemical, mechanical, thermal. It is believed that prostaglandins actually increase nociceptor sensitivity and thus heighten the response of nociceptors to the other chemical substances which activate nociceptors.

Initiation of an action potential

Once these chemicals are released, they cause a disturbance in the membrane potential of the nociceptor which causes a receptor potential. This in turn will initiate an action potential at the nociceptor–afferent fibre junction. An action potential is the passage of a wave of electrical charge along a nerve fibre membrane and it is the basis of how the nervous system transmits information. An action potential is an 'all or none' response, i.e. either it happens completely or it doesn't happen at all (see Ch. 3 for more detail on action potentials). Once the action potential is initiated, this is the start of activity in the ascending nociceptive pathways.

Afferent fibres

For most types of sensation, except that of smell, there are three types of neurones between the periphery and the cerebral cortex. They are:

- The first order neurone, which starts at the peripheral receptor and ends in the dorsal horn of the spinal cord.

• The second order neurone, which starts in the dorsal horn and terminates in the thalamus.
• The third order neurone, which starts in the thalamus and finishes in the sensory cortex.

The afferent fibres are therefore the first order neurones in the nociceptive pathways.

Nerve fibre classification system

There are two types of nerve fibre classification system in common use – an alphabetical system which has Aα, Aβ, A∂ and C fibres and a numerical system which has Groups I, II, III and IV fibre types. If the reader is not sure of the relationship between the two types of classification system, this can be confusing. For this reason, an approximate relationship between the alphabetical and numerical classification systems for sensory nerves is presented in Table 2.1. This text will adopt the numerical system as the main reference system but the alphabetical equivalent will also be provided in parentheses throughout the text so as to avoid any confusion.

Myelinated and unmyelinated fibres

The two types of afferent nerve fibres which transmit noxious information are the Group III (A∂) and Group IV (C) fibres. They are finely myelinated and unmyelinated respectively and thus conduct at comparatively slower speeds than the large diameter myelinated Group II (Aβ) fibres. Myelin is a lipid-like substance which forms a sheath around some nerve fibres, hence the term myelinated fibres; due to its presence,

these myelinated nerve fibres conduct faster than unmyelinated nerve fibres (see Ch. 3 for more detail). As the resistance to current flow in a nerve is inversely proportional to its diameter, it follows that small diameter nerve fibres (Groups III and IV) have a relatively high threshold for excitation compared to the large diameter fibres (Group II) which have a low threshold for excitation.

First and second pain

When an individual experiences pain, she can separate her experience into an initial sharp, fast type sensation and a latent slow, burning, aching type sensation. For example, if a person's finger is caught in a door, the initial pain is a sharp type which occurs immediately; after a couple of minutes this is replaced by a more burning, throbbing type of pain. These different types of pain are commonly referred to as first and second pain. Microneurographic studies have enabled neurophysiologists to establish that the first pain is transmitted by the Group III fibres and the second pain is transmitted by the Group IV fibres.

Dorsal horn

The cell bodies of Group III fibres and Group IV fibres lie in the dorsal root ganglia of the spinal cord. The central portion of these fibres enters the spinal cord in the lateral division of the dorsal root (approximately 15–20% of unmyelinated fibres enter via the ventral root and then travel to the dorsal horn). These fibres occupy the medial portion of Lissauer's tract; they bifurcate into ascending and descending branches which may travel for one to three segments before they synapse with second order neurones in the dorsal horn. Substance P is believed to be the neurotransmitter involved at the synapse between first and second order neurones. In the 1950s, Rexed discovered that the dorsal horn of the cat spinal cord could be segregated according to cytoarchitectural differentiation, into 10 segments or laminae (Rexed 1952). These laminae contain the cell bodies of second order neurones and receive

Table 2.1 Approximate relationships between the two types of sensory nerve fibre classification systems

Numerical	Alphabetical	Origin
Group Ia	Aα	Muscle spindles (annulospiral ending)
Group Ib	Aα	Golgi tendon organs
Group II	Aβ, Aγ	Touch/Pressure receptors Muscle spindles (flower-spray ending)
Group III	A∂	Temperature/Touch receptors/ Nociceptors
Group IV	C	Temperature/Touch receptors/ Nociceptors

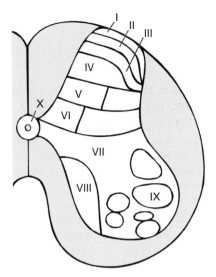

Figure 2.3 Arrangement of laminae in the grey matter of the spinal cord (after Rexed, 1952).

the axons of the incoming first order neurones (see Fig. 2.3). The incoming Group III and IV fibres synapse mainly in laminae I, II, III and V. Once they have synapsed, the second order neurones then cross to the opposite side of the spinal cord and ascend in one of two central pathways.

Spinal tracts/pathways

Some confusion can arise in ascribing names to the spinal tracts which carry the second order nociceptive neurones; this is primarily due to considerable variation and unnecessary complexity in the nomenclature adopted by several texts. The author prefers to keep this as straightforward as possible and thus the uncomplicated nomenclature suggested by Bond (1984) and Charman (1989) has been adopted for the current text. The two central pathways concerned with nociception are the lateral spinothalamic tract (LST) and the multisynaptic ascending system (MAS). Both have distinctive properties which make them easy to remember.

Lateral spinothalamic tract

This tract contains the second order neurones from Group III (A∂) fibres and thus carries the

first, sharp type pain. It is a fast conducting tract with relatively few collaterals (i.e. as it travels in the spinal cord, it does not have many synapses with other neural structures). The second order neurones in this tract end in the thalamus where they synapse with the nuclei of the ventrobasal complex.

Multisynaptic ascending system

As the name suggests, this is a diffuse system of many collaterals and relays throughout the brainstem. It carries the second order neurones from the Group IV (C) fibres and subsequently it carries the slow, burning, aching pain. The MAS second order neurones end by synapsing with the medial and intralaminar thalamic nuclei.

Second order neurones. Electrophysiological studies have identified two types of second order neurones which are involved in the transmission of noxious stimuli. One type is known as nociceptive specific (NS) neurones, whose cell bodies are located in lamina I of the dorsal horn and, as their name suggests, they are excited by nociceptive afferents. The second type of second order neurone is found in lamina V and responds to activity in Group II, III and IV fibres, hence they are termed wide dynamic range (WDR) neurones.

Brainstem structures

Several important brainstem structures are involved in the ascending nociceptive pathways and, additionally, in the descending modulation which arises due to activity in these pathways. Both of the ascending spinal pathways send collaterals (branches) to these structures; as previously mentioned, the MAS sends considerably more collaterals than the LST.

Reticular formation. The reticular formation (RF) is a diffuse network of neurones which extends from the medulla below to the thalamus above. The RF receives information from the majority of ascending sensory pathways and, in turn, it radiates information to different parts of the cerebral cortex; it is thus responsible for maintaining a state of alertness or awareness in the brain. It also influences motor control by sending signals to the descending motor pathways. With regard to nociception, it has a role in the affective-motivational aspects.

Periaqueductal grey matter and nucleus raphe magnus. The periaqueductal grey matter (PAG) and nucleus raphe magnus (NRM) are two important structures which play a role in the descending pain suppression system and opioid analgesia. Their involvement will be discussed in the next section (Neuromodulation of pain). Only a small proportion of fibres in the MAS ascend to the thalamus; the majority synapse in the reticular formation and thus have the effect of arousing the nervous system.

Thalamus

The thalamus consists of two masses of grey matter which are connected centrally and contain groups of nuclei. This important structure acts as a relay station for most types of sensation. At this stage of the ascending nociceptive pathways, nociception reaches the level of consciousness. The second order neurones which travelled in the two aforementioned spinal pathways terminate here in the ventrobasal, medial and intralaminar nuclei.

The ventrobasal complex receives neurones from the LST; the nuclei in this area of the thalamus are topographically arranged, i.e. points on different parts of the body relate directly to points in the nuclei. Third order neurones project to the primary sensory cortex where there is a similar topographical arrangement. The second order neurones in the MAS terminate in the medial and intralaminar nuclei which are not topographically arranged. The third order neurones from these nuclei project widely to the cerebral cortex, limbic system and basal ganglia.

It follows that information which passes through the MAS pathway can only be grossly localised compared to the accurate localisation of signals transmitted in the LST pathway.

Cerebral cortex

The final destination for nociception, and indeed all sensation, is the somatosensory cortex which is located in the post-central gyrus of the parietal lobe of the cerebral cortex. Here the perception and interpretation of sensation occurs. The somatosensory cortex defines the intensity, type and location of the sensation. An adjacent area of cortex, known as the association cortex, relates the sensation to past experience and memory. In the somatosensory cortex, the body is represented spatially according to the number of receptors in each body area. Areas which have a high density of receptors (e.g. the hand and lips) have a relatively large representative area, whereas the back has a smaller representation due to fewer receptors. This disparity gives rise to a distorted body image which is known as the sensory homunculus.

The limbic system. The limbic system consists of a number of interconnected structures which are located deep in the cerebral hemispheres. It has important connections with the hypothalamus and cerebral cortex and is involved in autonomic functions and the production of emotions. The limbic system is believed to play a role in the emotional aspects of pain.

NEUROMODULATION OF PAIN

The first section traced events in the ascending nociceptive pathways from the nociceptor in the periphery to the sensory cortex. We will now look at how the passage of nociceptive information may be interrupted at several stages along the ascending nociceptive pathways to produce neuromodulation of pain. Figure 2.4 divides the ascending pathways into four anatomical levels:

- peripheral
- spinal segmental
- supraspinal
- cortical.

Figure 2.5 illustrates the broad spectrum of physiotherapeutic modalities and techniques which are used to activate pain modulating mechanisms at each of the levels. A brief outline of the type of neuromodulation that occurs at each level is given below, followed by a more detailed explanation of those mechanisms specifically related to TENS analgesia.

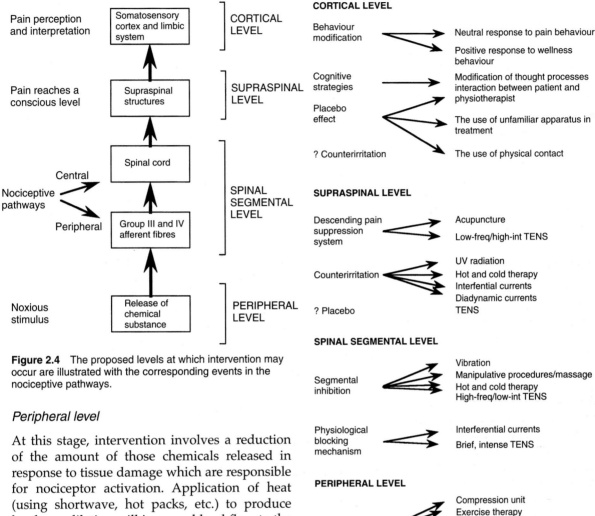

Figure 2.4 The proposed levels at which intervention may occur are illustrated with the corresponding events in the nociceptive pathways.

Figure 2.5 Examples of physiotherapeutic interventions at each of the four anatomical levels of the nociceptive pathways.

Peripheral level

At this stage, intervention involves a reduction of the amount of those chemicals released in response to tissue damage which are responsible for nociceptor activation. Application of heat (using shortwave, hot packs, etc.) to produce local vasodilation will increase blood flow to the affected area and it is therefore thought that this will assist in removing the chemicals. Other modalities (e.g. ultrasound), can affect cell permeability and thus reduce the amount of exudate formed in an inflammatory reaction. The pressure of exudate upon nociceptors can initiate activity in the nociceptive pathways; the application of ice immediately following tissue damage will produce local vasoconstriction and thereby reduce the pressure on nociceptors.

Spinal segmental level

Intervention at this stage involves the inhibition of activity in the small diameter Group III and

Group IV fibres before the incoming information ascends further up the neural axis. Segmental inhibition and physiological blocking, two mechanisms of neuromodulation which occur at this level, are discussed below (Mechanisms of neuromodulation) in more detail.

Supraspinal level

The ascending pathways make important synaptic connections with several brainstem structures involved with descending pain modulation systems. The placebo effect and counter-irritation are also believed to operate at this level.

Cortical level

At this level, intervention involves modification of the individual's perception and interpretation of pain. Behaviour modification and cognitive strategies are examples of psychological approaches which operate at this level.

MECHANISMS OF NEUROMODULATION RELEVANT TO TENS

The following sections discuss mechanisms of neuromodulation relevant to TENS analgesia in more detail.

Physiological blocking effect

Several in vivo and in vitro studies have reported that the application of high frequency electrical currents over a peripheral nerve reduces the conduction velocity of the nerve (Campbell & Taub 1973, Ignelzi & Nyquist 1976, 1979, Walmsley et al 1986; these studies are discussed in detail in Chapter 5). The recording of neural activity in a peripheral nerve before, during and after the application of TENS is the basic methodology employed in these studies. The easiest method of recording neural activity is by simply stimulating a nerve and recording the resultant compound action potential (CAP) using surface electrodes. A number of measurements can be obtained from the stored CAP, e.g. latency (from which velocity can be calculated), amplitude and area (see Ch. 5, Fig. 5.1).

In the study by Walmsley et al (1986), sensory CAPs were recorded from the human median nerve before any intervention, and a second set of CAPs were recorded after TENS electrodes were applied over the course of the nerve for 30 minutes but no current delivered. Finally, the TENS was delivered for 30 minutes and upon termination, a third set of CAPs were recorded. Analysis of the results showed that there was no significant difference in conduction velocity after the 30 minutes' application of TENS electrodes but there was a significant decrease in conduction velocity after the 30 minutes of TENS ($p = 0.003$). Skin temperature was also recorded from the index finger in this study; it was noted that temperature decreased significantly post TENS. Skin temperature is an important variable to consider in any nerve conduction experiment because conduction velocity varies with temperature. This study has therefore demonstrated that the application of TENS for 30 minutes can reduce the conduction velocity of afferent fibres.

In order to definitively identify which of the afferent fibre groups are affected by TENS, microneurographic studies are essential. Microneurographic recording techniques allow direct recording of electrophysiological activity from axons in peripheral nerves by means of small (tip < 5 μm), insulated, tungsten electrodes inserted directly into the nerve trunk (Kimura 1983). Such techniques allow selective recording of activity from different classes and types of afferents. Torebjörk & Hallin (1974) reported a progressive, frequency-dependent increase in latency of both A and especially C components of the radial nerve following repeated intradermal electrical stimulation (50–100 μs, 0.5–100 pulses/s).

The effect observed in the studies described above is believed to block activity primarily in the nociceptive fibres and thus has been referred to as a peripheral blockade of incoming nociceptive signals. Inherent in this mechanism is the assumption that when peripheral conduction is slowed, the volume of nociceptive traffic is reduced and this will reduce the overall perception of pain.

Segmental inhibition/gate control theory

The publication of the gate control theory of pain by Melzack & Wall (1965) served as a major impetus to the commercial production of TENS units for pain management. This theory produced the basic concept that stimulation of the large diameter (i.e. Group II) fibres (for example, by electrical currents) could reduce the perception of pain which resulted from activity in the small diameter fibres (Group III and IV). In the early 1970s, clinical evidence emerged which supported this theory (Wall & Sweet 1967); subsequently, the concept of electrical stimulation for pain relief was explored with renewed vigour. Despite the fact that the theory has since been disputed with regard to the precise location and mechanism involved in the 'gate', it is still held as a concept that some form of inhibition can occur by stimulation of large diameter afferents at a segmental level; hence the term 'segmental inhibition'.

The fundamental tenet of the theory is that a physiological gating mechanism exists in the dorsal horn of the spinal cord which may allow or inhibit nociceptive traffic to proceed centrally. Figure 2.6 shows the basic synaptic connections between the incoming afferents, the substantia gelatinosa (SG) and the 'T cell'. The T cell is believed to be a wide dynamic range type of second order neurone found in lamina V of the dorsal horn (see p. 15) which acts as a relay cell for ascending information. The relative amount of activity in the large and small diameter afferents determines whether or not the T cell relays the information further up the neuroaxis.

The substantia gelatinosa (lamina II and III) in the spinal dorsal horn, it is proposed, contains the gate. As indicated in Figure 2.6, the substantia gelatinosa has an inhibitory effect on the terminals of Group II, III and IV fibres which synapse with the T cell. The incoming fibres also have synaptic connections with the substantia gelatinosa; the small diameter Group III/IV fibres send an inhibitory collateral and the large diameter fibres send an excitatory collateral. Afferent information travelling in the Group II fibres will serve to increase the inhibitory effect of the SG upon the T cell and therefore close the gate to nociceptive traffic. Activity in the small diameter fibres reduces the inhibitory effect of the SG upon the T cell and therefore the gate is open and nociceptive traffic can proceed. There are also descending influences from a central control.

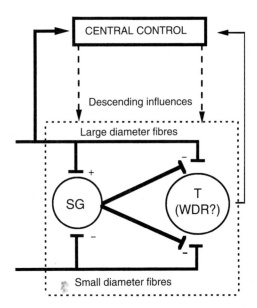

SG = substantia gelatinosa
WDR = wide dynamic range

Figure 2.6 Schematic diagram of the components of the 'gate' in the dorsal horn of the spinal cord.

Although the gate control model has been revised numerous times since its publication in 1965 and has lost much of original significance, it can still be viewed as a valuable contribution to neuroscience as it has provoked many questions on the physiological basis of nociceptive transmission. Professor Wall himself commented, several years after the publication of the theory, 'that a gate control exists is no longer open to doubt, but its functional role and its detailed mechanism remain open for speculation and for experiment' (Wall 1978).

Counterirritation

Counterirritation is a term used to describe intense somatic sensation applied to reduce pain. Counterirritants can be in the form of heat, cold or electrical therapy. It is believed that the intense sensory stimulation produced by counterirritation operates via a descending control system incorporated in the gate control theory.

Placebo effect

Clinicians tend to become offended if it is inferred that the principal mechanism of action of any therapeutic intervention they administer is the placebo effect – this should not be taken as a criticism. Is it not amazing that through touch, attention and listening skills alone, we can produce relief from the signs and symptoms of pain? Like any other modality that produces a sensation, TENS has placebo potential. The placebo effect has been reported to be as high as 30% in TENS analgesia (Thorsteinsson et al 1978). The patient–therapist interaction and the use of modalities have been described as important factors in the placebo effect.

The cognitive dissonance theory is one psychological explanation for placebo analgesia (Richardson 1994). This theory is based upon the fact that the patient has two beliefs which are psychologically inconsistent, which creates a state of tension (dissonance), e.g. they have received a treatment but they are not getting better. The patient may try to resolve this dissonance by altering their perception of their signs and symptoms.

The desire to get well to please the therapist is another psychological factor involved in placebo effect. It has also been suggested that placebo analgesia may occur due to the release of opioids (Basbaum & Fields 1984). The placebo response has been reported as varying from 0% to 100%, depending on the study cited (Wall 1992). Whatever the percentage, it must be acknowledged that therapists have in their hands a powerful tool which should be used to its maximum potential and not dismissed lightly.

Descending pain suppression system

One of the most productive areas of research during the past 2 decades has been the investigation of the role of opiates in the neuromodulation of pain. 'Opiates' is the collective name for compounds which are derivatives of the opium poppy and which include some of the most powerful analgesics available, the most commonly known being morphine. Although the psychopharmacological characteristics of morphine have been known for over a century, the existence of natural opiates (termed opioids) within the body has only been documented for the past 22 years; indeed, many of the precise functions and properties of opioids remain a topic for further deliberation and research. In the early 1970s, opiate receptors were identified in the brain, spinal cord and gastrointestinal tract. Hughes et al (1975) later discovered two naturally occurring opioid peptides, methionine- and leucine-enkephalin, which acted as agonists at opiate receptor sites. Within a few years, a number of other peptides were identified and now there are three known families of opioid peptides: enkephalin, dynorphin and β-endorphin. These peptides are commonly known as endorphins or endogenous opioids; this nomenclature refers to their endogenous morphine-like nature.

It has been established that a highly organised anatomical system for pain control exists which incorporates the endogenous opioids (Basbaum & Fields 1978, 1984). This system, referred to as the descending pain suppression system, is a three-tiered anatomical system which has the following principal components:

1. The periaqueductal grey matter (PAG), an area rich in opioid receptors.
2. The rostral ventral medulla (RVM) (the nucleus raphe magnus (NRM) and adjacent reticular nuclei).
3. The spinal dorsal horn.

Figure 2.7 illustrates the anatomical relationship of these three tiers.

Work by Reynolds (1969) and Mayer & Liebeskind (1974) demonstrated that stimulation of the PAG produced analgesia similar to that obtained with injecting doses of morphine into the same area; this analgesia was not accompanied by the behavioural depression observed with morphine and became known as stimulation produced analgesia (SPA).

Subsequent studies in humans demonstrated effective relief from clinical pain with SPA (Akil et al 1978, Hosobuchi et al 1977), and thus this discovery coincided with the discovery of endogenous opioids. Serotonin, noradrenaline and opioids are the important neurotransmitters in this descending system. Endogenous opioids

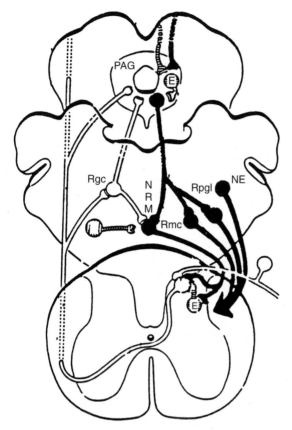

Figure 2.7 Schematic illustration of the major components of a descending system that contributes to the analgesic action of opiates and of electrical brain stimulation. The basic structure of the original model (Basbaum & Fields 1978) is retained. Highlighted in black are the connection between the projection neurones of the periaqueductal grey (PAG) and various subregions of the rostral ventral medulla (the nucleus raphe magnus (NRM), the nucleus reticularis magnocellularis (Rmc), and the nucleus reticularis paragigantocellularis lateralis (Rpgl)). The latter project via the dorsolateral funiculus to the spinal dorsal horn, where they inhibit nociceptive neurones. The inhibitory action at the cord may be via direct postsynaptic inhibition, or via an opioid peptide containing endorphin interneuron (indicated by stripes and 'E'). There are other endorphin links illustrated at the level of the PAG and the rostral medulla; however, their connections are not indicated. Inputs to the PAG (one of which is a hypothalamic B-endorphin pathway) are also illustrated as is the noradrenergic (NE) contribution to bulbospinal control. Finally, ascending components of this system are indicated by the unfilled symbols. These include afferent inputs (some of which are substance-P-containing) projection neurones of the dorsal horn, and their collaterals into the medulla and PAG. The ascending input to the PAG and raphe nuclei is presumed to derive, in part, from collaterals of neurones of the nucleus reticularis gigantocellularis (Rgc). (Reproduced, with permission, from the Annual Review of Neuroscience, Basbaum & Fields 1984, Volume 7, © 1984, by Annual Reviews Inc.)

are released at both brainstem and spinal cord levels. The net effect of opioid release at the level of the PAG and NRM is activation of descending projection neurones. Stimulation of the PAG by ascending fibres causes the release of opioids; it is believed that opioids released at this level have the effect of inhibiting an inhibitory interneurone and thereby excite the descending pathway to the NRM.

The RVM receives afferents from serotonin and neurotensin-containing neurones, thereby implying their role as neurotransmitters at this level (Fields & Basbaum 1989). RVM neurones project to the spinal dorsal horn via the dorso-lateral funiculus where the release of opioids has an inhibitory effect. It is believed that opioids bind to presynaptic receptor sites on substance P-containing nociceptive afferents and thus inhibit release of substance P; as substance P is a neurotransmitter necessary for nociceptive transmission this leads to the inhibition of the latter at a spinal cord level.

Summary

In summary, ascending nociceptive fibres send collaterals to the PAG which initiate activity in this system; PAG neurones project to the RVM where they have an excitatory influence. In turn, RVM neurones project to the spinal cord where they inhibit nociception. Acupuncture-like TENS is believed to operate primarily by this system through the stimulation of the small diameter afferents. This explains why analgesia associated with acupuncture-like TENS has a relatively longer onset latency compared to conventional TENS which operates primarily via local spinal segmental mechanisms. The longer latency is due to the considerable activity occurring in this complex system from the time of stimulation of the small diameter afferents to the final pre-synaptic inhibition at a spinal cord level.

In order to investigate the potential role of opioids in TENS analgesia, several studies have measured the level of endogenous opioids in blood plasma and cerebrospinal fluid before and after the application of TENS (Johnson et al 1992, O'Brien et al 1984, Salar et al 1981). The results of these studies remain equivocal; however, recent work has suggested that different modes of TENS induce differential release of opioid peptides (Han et al 1991, Han & Wang 1992).

THE PSYCHOLOGY OF PAIN – AN OVERVIEW

As already indicated above, pain is by definition a psychological phenomenon; thus no account of pain mechanisms would be complete without some review of the psychological substrates of pain. While this section provides a brief overview of the psychology of pain, it must be recognised that it cannot aim to be comprehensive nor exhaustive within the limits of the current text; for more in depth reviews, the reader is directed to more detailed texts such as Sternbach (1988).

Pain is experienced in an affected, cognitive and social context which is unique to the individual; as a consequence there is inherent variability between individuals in response to a given injury (essentially a fixed degree of nociceptive input). This variable link between injury and pain has been well recognised and represents in itself the most obvious evidence of the psychological basis of pain.

Pain causes changes in the individual's behaviour (i.e. their observable actions) which in the acute stage is essentially protective and facilitates healing and recovery. In the longer term, as the pain becomes chronic, such behaviours may predominate and no longer serve any useful purpose. Indeed, in some situations the 'pain behaviour' may be the cause of further disability, becoming an obstacle to rehabilitation and thus have to be specifically targeted for appropriate treatment. Such pain behaviours are various and may include poor posture, facial expressions such as grimacing, and alcohol or medication abuse. Where this is the case, any treatment plan should stress patient self-management with facilitation or reinforcement of appropriate ('well') behaviour together with negative reinforcement of the patient's pain behaviour.

Past experience influences pain and its associated behaviour; indeed, to a large degree, pain behaviour is essentially 'learned' (e.g. from parents) and conditioned by others through a variety of processes including direct instruction and observational learning. In addition to this, the emotional or affective context within which the injury or event causing pain arises for the individual will play a significant role in how that individual reacts to the injury and the associated pain. The nature of the pain experience is also affected by cognitive processes on the part of the individual or patient, e.g. attention, diversion or redefinition of the painful event, which may be facilitated as coping strategies.

Finally, the term psychogenic is frequently applied by health professionals to describe pain (or more appropriately pain behaviour) which is not commensurate with the objective organic findings or diagnosis; indeed, some may suggest that the patient's pain is not 'real'. In such cases it is important to remember, in the first instance, that all pains have a psychogenic element, as pain is ultimately a psychological phenomenon. Beyond this, it is important to realise that where the term 'psychogenic' is applied to reflect a lack of clinical findings, it is based on the assumption that diagnostic procedures are perfect (which is far from being the case), and thus does the patient a great disservice. For these reasons, it should be obvious that the question of whether a given patient's pain is 'real' is meaningless; for the patient, the pain is real and the objective for the health professional should be to treat that pain in the most appropriate way. To this extent, understanding how psychological factors influence an individual patient's pain experience will help the therapist in selecting and delivering the most effective treatment regime.

SUMMARY OF KEY POINTS

1. In this chapter, the author has discussed the key components in understanding the events which ultimately lead to the perception and also the modulation of the phenomenon of pain, which the poet John Milton succinctly described as 'the worst of all evils, an excessive, overturns all patience' (*Paradise Lost*, Book 6).

2. Pain is not a sensation, but rather a complex psychological and sensory experience which is

influenced by a number of other factors (e.g. social, cultural).

3. The principal components of the ascending pathways subserving the experience of pain are nociceptors, Group III and IV afferent fibres, spinal cord tracts (MAS and LST) and the somatosensory cortex.

4. The ascending nociceptive pathways can be divided into four levels at which the neuromodulation of pain may be achieved by a number of mechanisms. These levels are peripheral, spinal segmental, supraspinal and cortical.

5. The overall picture of the pain experience must also include the psychological aspects of pain.

REFERENCES

Akil H, Richardson D E, Hughes J, Barchas J D 1978 Enkephalin-like material elevated in ventricular cerebrospinal fluid of pain patients after analgetic focal stimulation. Science 201(4): 463–465

Basbaum A I, Fields H L 1978 Endogenous pain control mechanisms: review and hypothesis. Annals of Neurology 4: 451–462

Basbaum A I, Fields H L 1984 Endogenous pain control systems: brainstem spinal pathways and endorphin circuitry. Annual Review of Neuroscience 7: 309–338

Bond M R 1984 Pain: its nature, analysis and treatment, 2nd edn. Churchill Livingstone, Edinburgh

Campbell J N, Taub A 1973 Local analgesia from percutaneous electrical nerve stimulation. Archives of Neurology 28: 347–350

Charman R A 1989 Pain theory and physiotherapy. Physiotherapy 75(5): 247–254

Fields H L, Basbaum A I 1989 Endogenous pain control mechanisms. In: Wall P D, Melzack R (eds) Textbook of pain, 2nd edn. Churchill Livingstone, Edinburgh

Han J S, Wang Q 1992 Mobilization of specific neuropeptides by peripheral stimulation of identified frequencies. News in Physiological Sciences 7: 176–180

Han J S, Chen X H, Sun S L et al 1991 Effect of low- and high-frequency TENS on Met-enkephalin-Arg-Phe and dynorphin A immunoreactivity in human lumbar CSF. Pain 47: 295–298

Hosobuchi Y, Adams J E, Linchitz R 1977 Pain relief by electrical stimulation of the central gray matter in humans and its reversal by naloxone. Science 197: 183–186

Hughes J, Smith T W, Kosterlitz H W, Fothergill L A, Morgan B A, Morris H R 1975 Identification of two related pentapeptides from the brain with potent opiate agonist activity. Nature 258: 577–579

Ignelzi R J, Nyquist J K 1976 Direct effect of electrical stimulation on peripheral nerve evoked activity: implications in pain relief. Journal of Neurosurgery 45: 159–165

Ignelzi R J, Nyquist J K 1979 Excitability changes in peripheral nerve fibers after repetitive electrical stimulation. Journal of Neurosurgery 5: 824–833

Johnson M I, Ashton C H, Marsh V R, Thompson J W, Weddell A, Wright-Honari S 1992 The effect of transcutaneous electrical nerve stimulation (TENS) and acupuncture on concentrations of beta-endorphin,

met-enkephalin and 5-HT in the peripheral circulation. European Journal of Pain 13(2): 44–51

Kimura J 1983 Electrodiagnosis in diseases of nerve and muscle. Principles and practice. F A Davis, Philadelphia

Mayer D J, Liebeskind J C 1974 Pain reduction by focal electrical stimulation of the brain: an anatomical and behavioural analysis. Brain Research 68: 73–93

Melzack R, Wall P D 1965 Pain mechanisms: a new theory. Science 150: 971–979

Merskey H, Albe-Fessard A, Bonica J J et al 1979 Pain terms: a list with definitions and notes on usage. Pain 6: 249–252

O'Brien W J, Rutan F M, Sanborn C, Omer G E 1984 Effect of transcutaneous electrical nerve stimulation on human blood β-endorphin levels. Physical Therapy 64: 1367–1374

Reynolds D V 1969 Surgery in the rat during electrical analgesia induced by focal brain stimulation. Science 164: 444–445

Rexed B 1952 The cytoarchitectonic organization of the spinal cord in the cat. Journal of Comparative Neurology 96: 415–495

Richardson P H 1994 Placebo effects in pain management. Pain Reviews 1(1): 15–32

Salar G, Job I, Mingrino S, Bosio A, Trabucchi M 1981 Effect of transcutaneous electrotherapy on CSF β-endorphin content in patients without pain problems. Pain 10: 169–172

Sternbach J 1988 The psychology of pain. Raven Press, New York

Thorsteinsson G, Stonnington H H, Stillwell G K, Elveback L R 1978 The placebo effect of transcutaneous electrical stimulation. Pain 5: 31–41

Torebjörk H E, Hallin R G 1974 Excitation failure in thin nerve fiber structures and accompanying hypalgesia during repetitive electric skin stimulation In: Bonica J J (ed) Advances in Neurology. Raven Press, New York, Ch. 4, pp. 733–735

Wall P D 1978 The gate control theory of pain mechanisms: a re-examination and re-statement. Brain 101: 1–118

Wall P D 1992 The placebo effect: an unpopular topic. Pain 51(1): 1–3

Wall P D, Sweet W H 1967 Temporary abolition of pain in man. Science 155: 108–109

Walmsley R P, Monga T N, Prouix M 1986 Effect of transcutaneous nerve stimulation on sensory nerve conduction velocity: a pilot project. Physiotherapy Practice 2: 117–120

CHAPTER CONTENTS

Introduction 25

Physiology of nerve conduction 25
Membrane potentials 26
Development of membrane potentials 26
  The Nernst equation 27
Action potentials 27
Propagation of an action potential 28
  All or none principle 28
  Saltatory conduction 28
  Refractory period 29
Factors determining conduction velocity 29

Stimulation of a nerve using TENS 29
Strength–duration curve 30
Nerve fibre characteristics and stimulation
  parameters 30
Cathodal and anodal events 31
  Cathodal events 31
  Anodal events 31

Stimulation parameters of TENS 32
Types of current 32
Waveform 33
Frequency 33
Pulse duration 34
Intensity/amplitude 35

TENS – modes available 36
Conventional TENS 36
Acupuncture-like TENS 36
Burst train TENS 37
Brief, intense TENS 37
Continuous, burst and modulated outputs 37

Calibration of TENS units 37
  Calibration of pulse frequency 38
  Calibration of pulse duration 39
Measurement of the current output of a TENS
  unit 39
  Example 39

Summary of key points 40

3

TENS: physiological principles and stimulation parameters

INTRODUCTION

This chapter commences with an outline of the physiology of nerve conduction, which serves as a foundation for the ensuing description of how TENS initiates action potentials in a nerve. The stimulation parameters of TENS are outlined and subsequently the different types of TENS modes currently in use are discussed. Finally, a description of how to measure the pulse frequency, pulse duration and current output of a TENS unit is provided.

PHYSIOLOGY OF NERVE CONDUCTION

The basic structural unit of the nervous system is the nerve cell or neurone. The primary function of the nervous system is to convey information from one part of the body to another by the propagation of action potentials along neurones. Figure 3.1 illustrates the typical structure of a neurone; the central cell body usually has a number of processes called dendrites which carry information towards the cell body, and usually only one process which carries information away from the cell body called an axon (commonly referred to as a nerve fibre).

The section below gives an account of the development of membrane potentials and action potentials; for further detail the reader should refer to standard physiology textbooks (e.g. Ganong 1995, Guyton 1991, Schauf et al 1990).

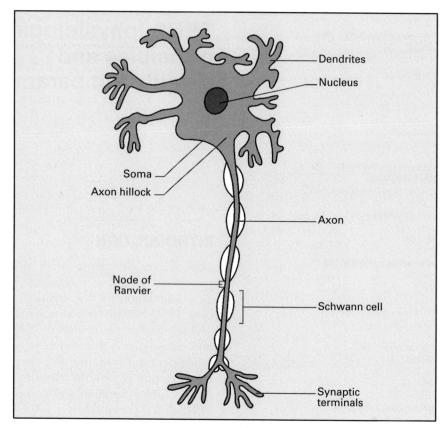

Figure 3.1 The structure of a typical neurone; the main components are a cell body (soma) and a number of processes (axon and dendrites).

Membrane potentials

Nerve cells have an electrical potential or charge across their membrane due to unequal concentrations of positive and negative ions in the intracellular and extracellular fluids (e.g. sodium (Na), potassium (K), calcium (Ca)). The magnitude of the resting membrane potential is –70 mV (i.e. the voltage difference which exits across the cell membrane when it is unstimulated), the inside being negatively charged with respect to the outside. The intracellular fluid contains large quantities of potassium (K⁺) and lower concentrations of sodium (Na⁺) and chloride (Cl⁻) relative to the extracellular fluid.

The resting nerve cell membrane is normally 50–100 times as permeable to potassium as to sodium, resulting in K⁺ diffusing with relative ease through the resting membrane but sodium diffusing only with difficulty. Within the intracellular fluid there are large numbers of negatively charged ions which either cannot diffuse at all or diffuse very poorly, e.g. protein and phosphate ions.

Development of membrane potentials

There are primarily two factors involved in the development of membrane potentials:

Sodium–potassium pump. The sodium–potassium pump is an active transport mechanism for sodium and potassium ions which is present in all cell membranes. This pump utilises adenosine triphosphate (ATP) as an energy source to actively transport K⁺ from outside to inside and Na⁺ from inside to outside. Normally, three Na⁺ ions are transported outside for every two

K+ ions transported inwards; this gives a net transfer of 50% more positive charges outward through the membrane than inward. This pump is called an electrogenic sodium–potassium pump because an electrical potential is created by its transport mechanism.

Ion concentration differences. The second means by which membrane potentials develop is the diffusion of ions through the cell membrane due to differences in the concentration of the ions. As there is a large sodium concentration gradient from outside to inside, the sodium ions tend to diffuse inwards creating positivity inside and negativity outside. The potassium ions diffuse outside creating negativity inside and positivity outside. Within milliseconds, the change in concentration of these ions causes the altered potential to block further diffusion of each of the ions across the membrane, i.e. when the sodium ions diffuse inwards creating electronegativity on the outside and electropositivity on the inside the potential difference tends to repel the inward flow of sodium ions.

The Nernst equation

The Nernst equation gives the relationship between the diffusion potential and the concentration difference of a particular type of ion. The membrane potential at which the electric force is equal in magnitude but opposite in direction to the concentration force is called the equilibrium potential for that ion.

$$E = \frac{-RT}{F} \log_{10} \frac{\text{Conc outside}}{\text{Conc inside}}$$

This equation is explained as follows:

E = equilibrium potential (mV). The equilibrium potential for sodium is +61 mV and –94 mV for potassium.

$\frac{RT}{F}$ = thermodynamic constants which have a value of $\approx$60 mV at body temperature

$\log_{10} \frac{\text{Conc outside}}{\text{Conc inside}}$

This is the log to the base 10 of the ratio of the concentration of the ion outside the membrane to the concentration of the ion inside the membrane.

Action potentials

Information is conveyed throughout the nervous system by the propagation of action potentials or 'nerve impulses'. Nerve and muscle cells are the only cell types capable of producing an action potential, An action potential results from rapid changes in the membrane permeability to potassium and sodium ions; this results in a short duration ($\approx$1 ms) alteration in membrane potential. In the rising phase of the action potential (see Fig. 3.2) the sodium permeability increases about 5000-fold and sodium ions then rush inwards. The loss of the normal negative potential inside the fibre by the influx of sodium ions is called depolarisation (i.e. the resting membrane potential becomes less negative). This is instantaneously followed by a return of the sodium permeability to normal and the potassium permeability increases greatly. Potassium ions now move to the outside because of their high concentration on the inside. This causes the membrane potential to return rapidly to its resting value which is known as repolarisation. The process of repolarisation therefore occurs due to the following:

- the increased sodium permeability is turned off (sodium inactivation)
- the membrane permeability to potassium increases.

During this phase of the action potential, the K+ permeability is even greater than during the resting state, which results in the membrane potential becoming even more negative than the resting membrane potential, i.e. –70 mV. This phase is known as after-hyperpolarisation (see Fig. 3.2).

The sodium and potassium concentrations are reestablished by the sodium–potassium pump. The sodium ions that diffused in and the potassium ions that diffused out are returned to their original state by the pump. This recharging process utilises energy derived from the ATP energy currency of the cell.

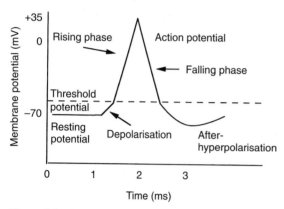

Figure 3.2 An action potential results from changes in the membrane potential.

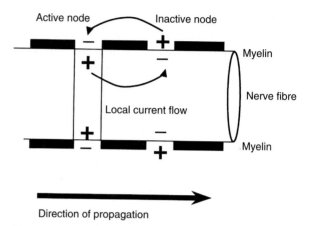

Figure 3.3 The spread of local current flow along a myelinated nerve fibre illustrates how an action potential is propagated.

Action potentials can only occur when the membrane is depolarised enough so that the sodium entry exceeds potassium efflux. The membrane potential at which this happens is called the threshold potential which is ≈5–15 mV more positive than the resting membrane potential. Many different types of stimuli, e.g. mechanical, electrical or thermal, have the ability to produce an action potential; they all do so by the same process, i.e. depolarisation of the membrane. However, it must be emphasised again that a stimulus, irrespective of its nature, will only be successful in initiating an action potential if the membrane potential is depolarised to the level of the threshold potential.

Propagation of an action potential

An action potential elicited at any one point on an excitable membrane will usually excite adjacent portions of the membrane, resulting in the propagation of the action potential. Each action potential triggers a new one at an adjacent area of membrane by local current flow (see Fig. 3.3). This local current flow occurs by positive ions moving from an area of relative positivity to an area of relative negativity; remember, like charges repel and unlike charges attract. If an action potential is initiated along the course of a nerve, it is propagated in both directions from its point of origin. However, physiological impulses arising from one end of an axon (the cell body or receptor) are conducted orthodromically

(orthodromic conduction is conduction in the normal physiological direction, i.e. central direction for a sensory neurone and peripheral direction for a motor neurone).

All or none principle

Regardless of the nature of the stimulus, the amplitude of the action potential generated is the same as long as depolarisation to the threshold level occurs. The 'all or none' property means that the action potential will either be maximal or will not occur at all.

Saltatory conduction

As an action potential is conducted along a nerve fibre, a certain amount of the local current generated will be lost by leakage between the nerve fibre and the surrounding environment. The presence of an insulating material would prevent such leakage and make the propagation of action potentials more efficient. Such an insulating material exists in the nervous system in the form of a myelin sheath. A myelinated nerve fibre is distinguished from an unmyelinated nerve fibre by the presence of a myelin sheath. A myelin sheath consists of many concentric layers of myelin wrapped around the axon, which functions as an insulator; the consistency of myelin is 80% lipid and 20% protein.

The myelin sheath is deposited around the axon by specialised cells called Schwann cells. The sheath is interrupted at intervals along its length by nodes of Ranvier, which are the junctions between two successive Schwann cells (this area between Schwann cells is uninsulated). Action potentials do not conduct along the sections of membrane protected by myelin, as the myelin electrically insulates the membrane. Thus, the action potential is conducted from node to node; this is known as saltatory conduction (*saltare* is the Latin for 'to leap'). This saltatory conduction not only conserves energy but also greatly increases the velocity of propagation of action potentials in myelinated fibres.

Refractory period

As long as the nerve fibre membrane is still depolarised from a preceding action potential, a second action potential cannot occur in an excitable fibre. This is due to the refractory period of the nerve; this is the period of time when a second action potential cannot be initiated by a stimulus which is normally large enough to cause depolarisation. This inability to depolarise is due to inactivation of the Na^+ channels.

The refractory period can be divided into two separate intervals – the absolute refractory period and the relative refractory period. The absolute refractory period is the interval of inexcitability which occurs immediately after the initiation of an action potential which lasts for $\approx 4 \times 10^{-4}$ ms in large myelinated nerve fibres. During the absolute refractory period, no stimulus will evoke a second action potential in the nerve fibre, no matter what intensities are used. Following the absolute refractory period there is a relative refractory period during which stronger than normal stimuli are required to excite the fibre; this lasts for 25% of the absolute refractory period.

The refractory period is inversely proportional to the conduction velocity of the nerve fibre. Large diameter nerve fibres (Group II/Aβ) will have short refractory periods due to their fast conduction rates; hence high electrical stimulation pulse frequencies can be used for stimu-

lation. In contrast, small diameter nerve fibres (Groups III/A∂ and IV/C) have relatively slower conduction rates and therefore longer refractory periods; hence much lower pulse frequencies are required for selective stimulation of these fibres.

Factors determining conduction velocity

The speed of propagation of action potentials is described in terms of the conduction velocity of the nerve. Velocity is defined as distance per unit time and is measured in metres per second (m/s). There are two important anatomical properties of nerve fibres which influence their conduction velocity:

- Diameter of the nerve. The propagation velocity of a nerve is directionally proportional to the diameter of the nerve. Large diameter fibres therefore conduct with faster velocities than small diameter fibres.
- Presence or absence of myelin. Conduction is much faster in myelinated fibres than non-myelinated fibres as the action potentials jump from one node of Ranvier to the next.

Other determinants of conduction velocity include (Kimura 1983):

- Faster rates of action potential generation which depolarise the adjacent segment more rapidly.
- Lower depolarisation thresholds of the cell membrane which allow the local current flow to depolarise the adjacent membrane in a shorter time.
- Higher temperatures which by increasing sodium conductance facilitate depolarisation.

STIMULATION OF A NERVE USING TENS

Having outlined the sequence of events involved in the initiation and propagation of an action potential, this section will now focus on the initiation of an action potential using an electrical current.

An external stimulus can cause depolarisation of a nerve and thus initiate an action potential

Table 3.1 Characteristics of sensory nerve fibres

Fibre type	Diameter (µm)	Conduction velocity (m/s)	Threshold for activation
Group II (Aβ)	12–20	30–120	Low
Group III (A∂)	1–4	5–15	High
Group IV (C)	< 1	0.2–2	High

as long as the stimulus depolarises the resting membrane potential to the threshold level. If the stimulus is electrical, as in TENS, the stimulation parameters of frequency, pulse duration and intensity must correlate with the characteristics of the nerve fibre itself. Table 3.1 summarises the characteristics of Group II, III and IV afferent fibres. Group II fibres carry primarily touch and pressure information whereas the other two groups carry nociceptive information (see Ch. 2 for further detail).

Strength–duration curve

The relationship between the stimulation parameters of pulse amplitude and duration of the stimulating current can be illustrated on a strength–duration (SD) curve. Basically, this curve illustrates the relationship between different combinations of pulse duration and amplitude which are required to optimally stimulate a given fibre type and produce the response associated with the fibre, i.e. motor, sensory or noxious response. Figure 3.4 illustrates strength–duration curves for motor, sensory and nociceptive fibres. Note that at any given pulse duration, the order of recruitment with increasing stimulus amplitude is first sensory, then motor, then nociceptive fibres. At the shorter pulse durations, the separation between the three curves becomes greater, indicating easier differentiation between the three fibre types.

The SD curve itself is an indicator of the threshold required to cause depolarisation of a given nerve fibre type. A subthreshold stimulus will have parameter combinations that fall to the left of the SD curve and will therefore not initiate an action potential. A suprathreshold stimulus will have parameter combinations that fall to

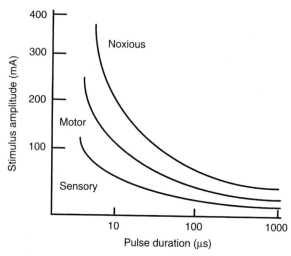

Figure 3.4 Strength–duration curves for sensory, motor and noxious responses. Any stimulus which has a combination of pulse amplitude and pulse duration which falls to the left of a specified curve is regarded as subthreshold and will not initiate an action potential. A stimulus which has a combination of pulse amplitude and pulse duration which falls to the right of a specified curve is regarded as suprathreshold and will initiate an action potential to produce the particular response specific to the type of nerve, i.e. motor, sensory.

the right of the curve and will initiate an action potential.

If an electrical stimulus is applied over a mixed nerve, the order of response is first sensory (Group II/Aβ fibres); the patient will report a sensation of paraesthesia (pins and needles) as a result of external stimulation of these fibres. The motor fibres are recruited next, with associated contractions, and finally nociceptive (Group III/A∂ and IV/C) fibres are stimulated which evoke a painful response.

Nerve fibre characteristics and stimulation parameters

Most peripheral nerves are mixed (i.e. they contain a combination of both motor and sensory fibres). Consequently, when an electrical stimulus is applied over a mixed nerve, the individual characteristics of the component fibres will determine which fibres are stimulated. The inner longitudinal resistance to current flow in a nerve fibre varies inversely with the diameter of the nerve fibre; therefore the large diameter Group II (Aβ) fibres have a low threshold for activation, in that low current intensities are required to depolarise the resting membrane potential to the threshold level. Group II fibres conduct relatively fast and therefore have short refractory periods; it has been observed that high stimulation frequencies are effective for stimulation. From the strength–duration curve (Fig. 3.4) one can see that a short pulse duration is required to selectively activate these fibres. In summary, selective activation of Group II fibres requires a stimulus with a low intensity, high frequency and a short pulse duration.

In contrast, Group III (A∂) and IV (C) fibres conduct relatively slowly and have relatively longer refractory periods, therefore it is more appropriate to use a low pulse frequency. If a current with a high pulsing frequency were applied to this fibre type it would not cause initiation of successive action potentials because the nerve fibre would not have recovered sufficiently from the previous action potential. These fibres have high threshold values due to their small diameter and therefore high stimulus intensities are required for stimulation. Finally, the strength–duration curve (discussed above) indicates that longer pulse durations are desirable for selective stimulation. In summary, Group III and IV fibres require a stimulus with a low frequency, high intensity and long pulse duration for selective stimulation.

One can see that the individual characteristics of the different types of nerve fibres are used to determine the stimulation parameters required to provide an adequate stimulus to initiate an action potential in the respective nerve fibre.

Cathodal and anodal events

In a TENS electrode circuit, one electrode is positively charged (anode) and the other negatively charged (cathode) (see section below, 'Waveform', for monophasic and biphasic waveforms). Figure 3.5 illustrates the current flow between two TENS electrodes applied to the skin; as the arrows indicate, the current flows from anode to cathode. Figures 3.6a and 3.6b illustrate the changes in membrane potential which occur under the cathode and anode electrodes respec-

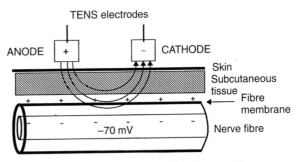

Figure 3.5 Schematic representation of current flow through the skin between two TENS electrodes.

tively. It is important to bear in mind that one of the principles of electric charge is that like charges will repel and unlike charges will attract, therefore the same will apply to positive and negative ions. In the following account, it is easier to focus on the events which occur in terms of negatively charged ions.

Cathodal events

The cathode electrode is negatively charged. As depolarisation of the nerve membrane occurs under the cathode, it is therefore commonly termed the active electrode. As the electrical current flows from anode to cathode, negative charges tend to accumulate on the outer surface of the nerve fibre membrane as they will be repelled by the negatively charged cathode; this makes the outside of the nerve fibre membrane relatively more negative. Consequently, the inside of the membrane becomes more positive due to the accumulation of positive ions on the inside. Because of these events, the resting membrane potential will change towards a more positive value, i.e. depolarisation occurs. Remember that depolarisation is the loss of the normal negative value of the resting membrane potential.

Anodal events

The reverse occurs under the positively charged anode; negative charges tend to move from the outside of the membrane towards the anode because they are attracted to the positive charge of the anode. This makes the outside of the

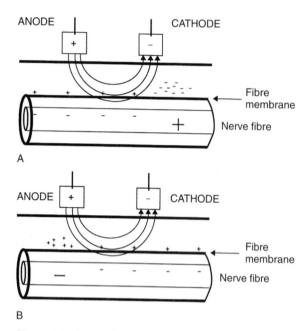

Figure 3.6 Current flowing between the two electrodes causes (A) depolarisation under the negative electrode (cathode) and (B) hyperpolarisation under the positive electrode (anode).

membrane relatively more positive, which has the effect of making the inside potential more negative and so hyperpolarisation occurs here. Hyperpolarisation is the change in membrane potential towards a more negative value.

Once the critical level of depolarisation occurs (i.e. threshold level is reached), an action potential is initiated. As indicated before, an action potential initiated along the course of a nerve will propagate in both directions.

STIMULATION PARAMETERS OF TENS

This section briefly outlines the stimulation parameters of TENS and is followed by a description of the four different modes of TENS, which basically consist of different combinations of these parameters.

Types of current

There is considerable confusion in current texts regarding the accurate description of TENS in

terms of type of current; for example, some sources say TENS is a modified direct current (DC), whereas others refer to it as a pulsed current. Figure 3.7 illustrates the three basic types of electrotherapeutic current which can be described as follows:

1. Direct current (DC). A direct current is one in which unidirectional current (i.e. in one direction only) flows continuously over time.

2. Alternating current (AC). An alternating current is one in which bidirectional current (i.e. in both directions) flows continuously over time.

3. Pulsed current. A pulsed current is one in which the unidirectional or bidirectional flow of current periodically ceases over time.

From these descriptions, and from Figure 3.7, it can be logically concluded that it is most accurate to describe TENS as a pulsed current and not as AC or DC. This brings us on to the next parameter – waveform.

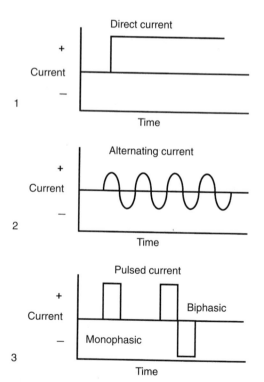

Figure 3.7 The three basic types of electrotherapeutic current – DC, AC and pulsed current. The graphs illustrate the changes in the direction of current over time.

Waveform

The waveform of a current simply refers to its shape as seen on a graph of amplitude versus time. A monophasic waveform means that current flows in only one direction (see Fig. 3.7), therefore one electrode acts as the cathode (negative) and the other as the anode (positive). A biphasic waveform means that current flows in both directions, thus each electrode acts as a cathode for some part of the waveform. The waveform therefore has two components (or phases), a positive and a negative component which represent the change in current flow.

A waveform is termed symmetrical if the portion of the waveform in the first phase is an exact mirror image but opposite in direction to the portion of the waveform in the second phase (i.e. current flow is equal in magnitude and duration in both directions). A biphasic symmetrical waveform results in each electrode acting as a cathode (i.e. the active electrode) during alternate phases of the pulse. In contrast, an asymmetrical biphasic waveform has two phases which are not equal in shape (i.e. the duration and magnitude of current flow is not equal in both directions). Due to this inequality, this typically means that only one direction of current flow (i.e. one phase of the waveform) is adequate to cause depolarisation and therefore this waveform acts like a monophasic waveform in that only one electrode acts as the active electrode.

TENS waveforms are usually described as asymmetrical biphasic rectangular or symmetrical biphasic rectangular; Figure 3.8 illustrates three typical TENS waveforms.

TENS waveforms usually have a zero net DC;

this means that the amount of charge under the positive portion of the waveform is equal to the amount of charge under the negative portion of the waveform. The production of a zero net DC reduces the likelihood of chemical skin irritation; a direct current can potentially cause skin irritation due to the build up of ions of one charge under the electrodes.

Frequency

Frequency is a time-dependent characteristic which is measured in hertz (Hz). The frequency of a current refers to the number of pulses delivered per second – a frequency of 150 Hz means that 150 pulses are delivered per second. Figure 3.9 illustrates how the frequency of an alternating current and a pulsed current can be calculated. In each case, the frequency is calculated using the following equation:

$$\text{Frequency} = \frac{1 \text{ second}}{\text{period}}$$

The period is the time elapsed between a specific point on the waveform of the pulse to the identical point on the next pulse. The period of the waveform in an alternating current is the time taken for the current to flow in one direction and then back in the other direction (i.e. the time taken for one complete cycle). In the example given, the frequency is 1 s divided by 250 μs (125 μs + 125 μs) which equals 4000 Hz. For a pulsed current, the period is the pulse duration plus the interpulse duration (the time elapsed between pulses). In the example given, the frequency is 1 s divided by 5 ms (2 ms + 3 ms) which equals 200 Hz.

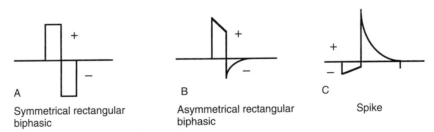

A	B	C
Symmetrical rectangular biphasic	Asymmetrical rectangular biphasic	Spike

Figure 3.8 Examples of three common TENS waveforms; each has a zero net DC component.

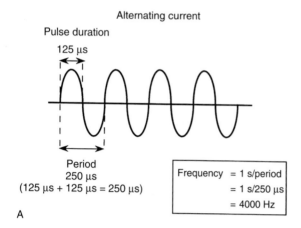

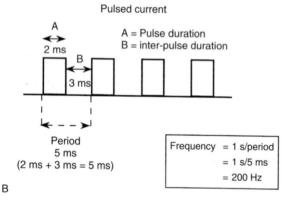

Figure 3.9 The frequency of a current equals 1 s divided by the period. The period is the time elapsed between one specific point on the waveform to the the identical point on the next waveform. Examples are given for frequency calculations for both an alternating current and a pulsed current.

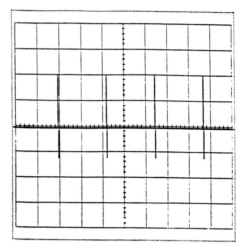

Low frequency TENS current (4 Hz)
Sweep duration = 100 ms per division

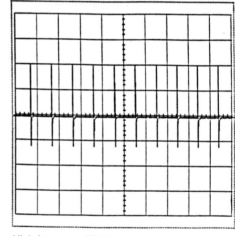

High frequency TENS current (100 Hz)
Sweep duration = 10 ms per division

Figure 3.10 Oscilloscope traces illustrating a low and a high frequency TENS current.

Figure 3.10 is a print-out from an oscilloscope to illustrate examples of both low and high frequency stimuli. Typically, the frequency range of most commercially available TENS units is 0–200/250 Hz. Some manufacturers use the term 'rate' rather than frequency to indicate the frequency dial/control.

Pulse duration

This parameter is another time-dependent characteristic, also commonly referred to as pulse width. The unit of pulse duration is usually given in microseconds (μs), which is a unit of time, hence it is more correct to use the term 'duration' rather than 'width'. Indeed, some confusion surrounds the exact portion of the waveform that the pulse duration refers to. Some texts refer to the phase duration as the duration of the waveform that is either positive (positive phase) or negative (negative phase) and thus subsequently refer to the pulse duration as the duration of both phases in the waveform, i.e. the sum of the duration of both positive and negative phases. How-

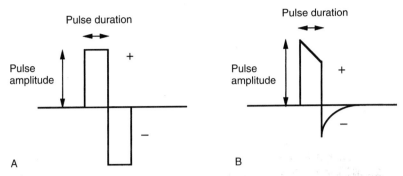

Figure 3.11   Pulse duration and amplitude parameters.

ever, most texts tend to refer to the pulse duration as the duration of only the positive component of the waveform as indicated in Figure 3.11 and this text will adhere to this definition. Figure 3.12 is an oscilloscope print-out of two TENS waveforms with short and long pulse durations. TENS pulse durations are in the μs range (1 μs = 1×10^{-6} s). If the pulse duration is quoted in terms of milliseconds (ms), it is useful to know that 100 μs = 0.1 ms.

Intensity/amplitude

Intensity refers to the magnitude of current or voltage applied by the unit and can be measured in milliamps (mA) or volts (V) respectively. Current is the flow of electric charge and voltage is the driving force required to move this electric charge; it should be remembered that it is the level of the current and not the voltage that is ultimately responsible for depolarisation of a nerve fibre membrane.

The relationship between current and voltage is provided by Ohm's law:

$V = IR$

where V is the voltage required to move an electric charge (I) across a resistance (R) which opposes the movement of electric charge. When an electrical current is applied to the skin it will require a driving force because it will encounter impedance (resistance) in the electrode–patient system (in a TENS unit the driving force is supplied by the battery).

The reader should be aware that TENS units are typically designed with a constant current or

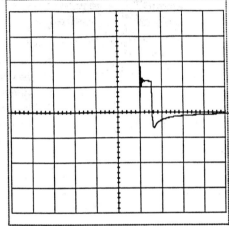

A

Short pulse duration TENS current (50 μs)
Sweep duration = 100 μs per division

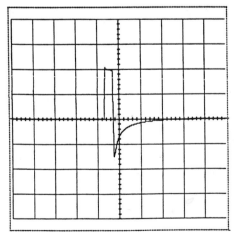

B

Long pulse duration TENS current (200 μs)
Sweep duration = 500 μs per division

Figure 3.12   Oscilloscope traces illustrating a short and a long pulse duration TENS current.

constant voltage output, which means that either the voltage or current (respectively) will vary to maintain a constant current or voltage amplitude (within limits) as the impedance of the electrode–patient system changes (impedance is discussed in greater detail in Ch. 4). The intensity of a constant current unit is measured in milliamps and the intensity of a constant voltage unit is measured in volts.

It is important to note that there is not necessarily a linear relationship between the intensity dial settings on a TENS unit and the actual amplitude of stimulation, i.e. similar increments of the intensity dial do not necessarily increase the amplitude by equivalent amounts. Figure 3.13 shows an intensity dial calibration curve with a 1 kΩ load for a standard TENS unit. This is a graph of the intensity dial settings of 1–10 plotted against the voltage recorded from an oscilloscope (see p. 39 on how to do this). The graph clearly illustrates the non-linear nature of intensity alteration, i.e. an intensity setting of 4 will not necessarily produce twice the stimulation amplitude at a setting of 2. This has very important implications in that small changes of the intensity dial could result in the patient experiencing dramatic sensory changes. Similarly, it should be pointed out that the actual frequency and pulse

duration settings on a machine are not necessarily the same as the value indicated by the manufacturer (see Ch. 4, Fig. 4.3). Therefore, if a TENS unit is used for a piece of research, either experimental or clinical, it is imperative that the parameters are calibrated on an oscilloscope (see p. 37 for calibration of a TENS unit).

TENS – MODES AVAILABLE

There are currently four TENS modes used in clinical practice. Any commercially available unit should provide the necessary parameter ranges to allow all four modes to be set on the same unit (this requires variable frequency, pulse duration and intensity settings and burst versus continuous output).

Conventional TENS

Conventional (or high frequency / low intensity) TENS is the most commonly used mode of TENS. The stimulation parameters are as follows:

- a low intensity
- a high frequency, typically above 100 Hz
- the pulse duration is usually short (50–80 μs).

This combination of parameters stimulates the Group II (Aβ) afferents (see p. 30 for characteristics). The sensation experienced with conventional TENS is one of comfortable paraesthesia with no muscle contractions, although if the electrodes are placed over a motor point, some contraction is visible with higher stimulation intensities. As the Group II fibres are stimulated, this TENS mode achieves analgesia primarily by spinal segmental mechanisms, i.e. gating effects. Thus the analgesia is of relatively rapid onset because local neurophysiological mechanisms are responsible; however, the analgesia tends to be relatively short, typically lasting only for up to a few hours post treatment.

Acupuncture-like TENS

It is a common misconception that this mode derived its name from application over acupuncture points. Acupuncture-like (or low frequency /

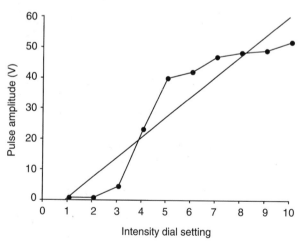

Figure 3.13 Graph of intensity dial settings plotted against recorded voltage for a TENS unit; the straight line indicates a true linear relationship. This TENS unit clearly does not have a linear relationship between intensity settings and amplitude.

high intensity) TENS primarily stimulates the Group III (A∂) and IV (C) nociceptive fibres and small motor fibres. The stimulation parameters are:

- a low frequency (usually 1–4 Hz)
- a high intensity (high enough to produce visible muscle contractions)
- a long pulse duration (~200 μs).

The electrodes should be positioned to produce visible muscle contractions, e.g. over a myotome related to the painful area. The patient will experience paraesthesia and muscle contraction (twitching type) with this mode. As muscle contractions occur, additional sensory information is carried from the muscle spindle via muscle afferents. It is desirable that the patient experiences motor contraction, therefore the intensity should be increased until the patient feels this. This mode of TENS is believed to operate primarily through the descending pain suppression system (see Ch. 2); thus there is a relatively longer onset to analgesia but the analgesia typically lasts longer than with conventional TENS.

Burst train TENS

Some texts refer to this next mode of TENS as acupuncture-like TENS; the main difference in definition is that the burst train mode has high frequency trains of pulses delivered at a low frequency, whereas the mode described in the last section has single pulses delivered at a low frequency. This burst train mode of TENS is really a mixture of conventional and acupuncture-like TENS, and comprises a baseline low frequency current together with high frequency trains. Typically, the frequency of the trains is 1–4 Hz with the internal frequency of the trains around 100 Hz. This type of TENS was developed by Eriksson & Sjölund (1976) as a result of their experiences with Chinese electroacupuncture. They found that when high frequency trains of electrical stimuli were delivered at a low frequency via an acupuncture needle, patients could tolerate the stimulus intensity required to produce the desired strong muscle twitches much better than when single impulses were delivered through the needle (the authors refer

to this mode as acupuncture-like TENS). Some patients prefer this mode to acupuncture-like TENS because the pulse trains produce a more comfortable muscle contraction.

Brief, intense TENS

This mode of TENS uses a high frequency (100–150) Hz, long pulse duration (150–250 μs) at the patient's highest tolerable intensity for short periods of time (< 15 minutes). Mannheimer & Lampe (1984) recommend that this mode can be used for painful procedures such as skin debridement, suture removal, etc.

Continuous, burst and modulated outputs

Most TENS units offer variable intensity, pulse duration and frequency settings. In addition, another switch may be available which will allow the user to choose between continuous, burst and modulated outputs (see Fig. 3.14). The continuous and burst outputs are self-explanatory, the latter is used in burst train TENS as described above. The modulated output means that there is a variation in either pulse duration, frequency or amplitude parameters in a cyclic fashion. Indeed, some units have modulation of two or all three of these parameters. If the output is set for amplitude modulation (see Fig. 3.14), a cyclic modulation in amplitude is produced which increases from zero to a preset level then back to zero again. This choice of modulated output has been included by manufacturers to overcome accommodation of nerve fibres and to provide more comfort to the patient; the reality of this remains debatable, although some experimental pain work has been completed comparing this output to others (Johnson et al 1991).

CALIBRATION OF TENS UNITS

The previous sections have described the stimulation parameters of TENS. As indicated earlier, the settings on a TENS unit are not always accurately marked. These settings can be checked and altered (i.e. calibrated) quite easily if one has access to an oscilloscope. In order to calibrate

Continuous
output

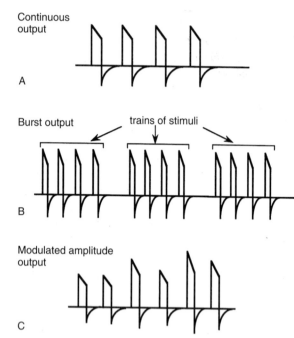

Burst output   trains of stimuli

Modulated amplitude
output

Figure 3.14 Illustration of continuous, burst and modulated types of output available on most TENS units.

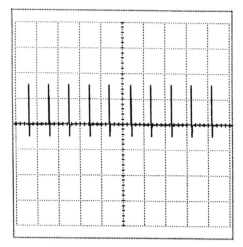

A

Calibration of 100 Hz frequency. Sweep duration of the oscilloscope = 10 ms per division. Time represented by the entire screen is 10 squares × 10 ms = 100 ms (0.1 s). The frequency dial of the TENS is adjusted to display 10 pulses on the screen; if 10 pulses appear in 0.1 s, therefore in 1 second there would be 100 pulses, i.e. the frequency = 100 Hz.

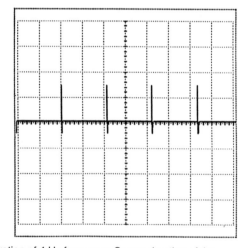

B

Calibration of 4 Hz frequency. Sweep duration of the oscilloscope = 100 ms per division. Time represented by the entire screen is 10 squares × 100 ms = 1000 ms (1 second). The frequency dial of the TENS is adjusted to display 4 pulses on the screen; as there are 4 pulses in 1 second therefore the frequency = 4 Hz.

Figure 3.15 Oscilloscope traces illustrating calibration of 100 Hz and 4 Hz frequency.

either pulse frequency or duration, some basic knowledge of the operation of an oscilloscope is required.

The first step is to attach the two TENS electrode leads to the leads of the oscilloscope and obtain a display of the TENS waveform on the oscilloscope screen by altering the voltage sensitivity and sweep duration settings. Then follow the procedures outlined below for calibration of pulse frequency or pulse duration. This can be done purely to check the manufacturer's settings at regular intervals or as part of a calibration process for a clinical or experimental study where it is very important that accurate calibration of equipment is carried out. Figures 3.15 and 3.16 show oscilloscope traces of a TENS waveform used to calibrate the pulse frequency and duration parameters given in the following examples.

Calibration of pulse frequency

If you are calibrating a high frequency (e.g. 100 Hz), set the sweep duration of the oscilloscope so that

the time represented by the entire screen is $\frac{1}{10}$ of a second (i.e. 0.1 s). Then alter the frequency dial on the TENS so that the number of pulses/waveforms visible on the oscilloscope screen is $\frac{1}{10}$

of your frequency value; in this case $\frac{1}{10}$ of 100 (100 Hz) is 10, therefore 10 pulses should be visible (Fig. 3.15).

If you are calibrating a low frequency, e.g. 4 Hz, then alter the sweep duration of the oscilloscope so that the time represented by the screen is 1 second. Then alter the frequency dial to display only four pulses/waveforms (Fig. 3.15B).

Calibration of pulse duration

Alter the sweep duration of the oscilloscope to display one pulse/waveform. Most oscilloscopes have a function so that if you place two cursors either side of the pulse, the oscilloscope can automatically calculate the pulse duration. If this function is not available, an alternative method is simply to count up the number of full squares or portion of a full square on the oscilloscope screen that the positive part of the waveform occupies (see Fig. 3.16). Therefore, if each square represents 50 µs and the positive part of the pulse occupies 2.5 squares, the pulse duration is $2.5 \times 50\ \mu s = 125\ \mu s$.

Measurement of the current output of a TENS unit

The current output of a TENS unit at each intensity setting can also be measured using an oscilloscope. As skin–electrode impedance (resistance) should be taken into account, the TENS leads are connected across a resistor. The leads of an oscilloscope are connected to each end of the resistor to measure the voltage drop across it (see Fig. 3.17). A 1 kΩ resistor is usually used as this is taken to approximately represent the average skin–electrode impedance (Roth & Wolf 1978). Once the TENS waveform is obtained on the oscilloscope screen, a cursor can be used to measure the height of the positive part of the waveform which represents the voltage. If a cursor is not available on the oscilloscope, then the number of squares or portion of squares that the height of the positive part of the waveform occupies can be counted. This latter method is not as accurate as the first. As the voltage and the resistance are now known, the value of the current can be calculated using Ohm's law as illustrated in the example below.

Example

At an intensity setting of 5 on a TENS unit, the voltage measured across a 1 kΩ resistor is 39.2 V. What is the current output at this setting?

$V = 39.2\ V$ $V = IR$
$R = 1\ k\Omega = 1000\ \Omega$
$I = ?$ $I = \dfrac{V}{R}$

$$I = \frac{39.2}{1000} = 0.039\ A$$
$$= 3.9\ mA$$

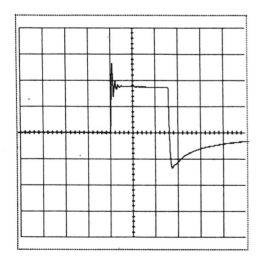

Figure 3.16 Oscilloscope trace illustrating calibration of 125 µs pulse duration. Sweep duration of the oscilloscope = 50 µs per division. The positive part of the waveform (i.e. pulse duration) occupies 2.5 squares, therefore pulse duration is $2.5 \times 50\ \mu s = 125\ \mu s$.

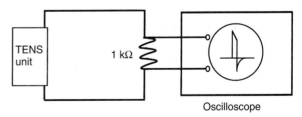

Figure 3.17 Circuit diagram used for measurement of current output of a TENS unit. The voltage across a 1 kΩ resistor is obtained from the oscilloscope.

By recording the voltage for each intensity dial setting, the current output at each dial setting can be calculated using the above method.

These calibration procedures are not difficult to do and can be easily incorporated into a routine checking procedure of electrotherapy apparatus in an outpatients department or private clinic. It is imperative that a TENS unit is calibrated accurately before embarking on a clinical trial in order to ensure the reliability of the results.

SUMMARY OF KEY POINTS

1. The nervous system communicates information by the propagation of action potentials along neurones. Action potentials are transient changes in the resting membrane potential of neurones.

2. Neurones can be stimulated/excited by the external application of electrical currents.

3. An electrical stimulus must have certain characteristics which are compatible with those of the nerve to be stimulated in order for an action potential to be elicited.

4. There are four modes of TENS used; all TENS units should allow manipulation of stimulation parameters to produce all four modes.

REFERENCES

Eriksson M, Sjölund B 1976 Acupuncture-like electroanalgesia in TNS-resistant chronic pain. In: Zotterman Y (ed) Sensory functions of the skin in primates. Pergamon Press, Oxford
Ganong W F 1995 Review of medical physiology, 17th edn. Prentice-Hall, London
Guyton A C 1991 Textbook of medical physiology, 8th edn. W B Saunders, Philadelphia
Johnson M I, Ashton C H, Bousfield D R, Thompson J W 1991 Analgesic effects of different pulse patterns of transcutaneous electrical nerve stimulation on cold-induced pain in normal subjects. Journal of Psychosomatic Research 35(2/3): 313–321
Kimura J 1983 Electrodiagnosis in diseases of nerve and muscle: principles and practice. F A Davis, Philadelphia
Mannheimer J S, Lampe G N 1984 Clinical transcutaneous electrical nerve stimulation. F A Davis, Philadelphia
Roth M G, Wolf S L 1978 Monitoring stimulation parameters from clinical transcutaneous nerve stimulators. Physical Therapy 58(5): 586–587
Schauf C L, Moffett D F, Moffett S B 1990 Human physiology: foundations and frontiers. Times Mirror/ Mosby College Publishing, St Louis

CHAPTER CONTENTS

Introduction   41

The TENS unit   41
Constant current or constant voltage   44

**The electrical properties of the electrode–skin
    interface   45**
The electrode–gel–skin interface   45
The electrode–gel interface   45
    Polarisation   47
    Electrode materials   48

The skin   48
Structure of the skin   48
Electrical properties of the skin   49
    The skin's parallel capacitance (C_{SP})   50
    The skin's parallel resistance (R_{SP})   51
    Electrode gels and their effects   51
    Electrode and skin preparation   52
Overall impedance   53
Importance of electrode–skin impedance   53
Current density   54
Skin irritation   55

TENS electrodes   57
Electrode size and shape   57
Electrode attachment   58
Electrode design   59

Summary of key points   61

4

Basic electronic and electrode principles

INTRODUCTION

This chapter deals with some of the basic principles associated with TENS units and, in particular, the electrodes. The construction and function of a basic TENS unit are described and the advantages/disadvantages of using constant current or constant voltage impulses are compared. The electrical properties of the various components of the electrode–gel–skin interface are studied with a view to imparting a basic understanding of the underlying principles. Methods of optimising the electrical properties of the electrode–skin interface are presented. Finally, all of the above aspects are brought together in a section on electrode design. It is anticipated that the reader will then be in a better position to decide which electrode is best for a given application.

THE TENS UNIT

A basic TENS unit comprises a power source, an oscillator stage and an amplifier stage. The various component parts of the stimulator can be powered by either batteries (DC) or mains electricity (AC). A simple block diagram of a TENS device is shown in Figure 4.1. Most systems are battery powered for portability and safety. When the input is a mains AC voltage, the large amplitude signal (240 V in the UK; 115 V in the USA) must first be changed into a lower amplitude DC voltage. In the case of a battery-powered device, one already starts with a DC voltage. However, as batteries can only generate relatively low DC

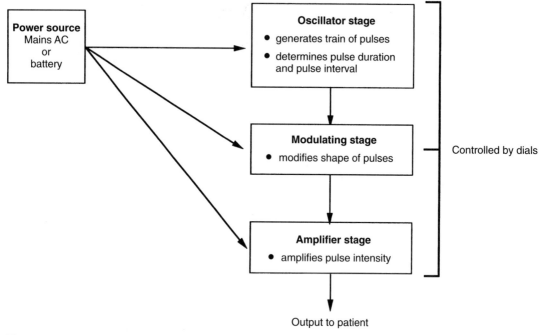

Figure 4.1 Block diagram of the inside of a TENS unit. (After Low & Reed, 1994.)

voltages, usually in the range of 1.5 to 9 V, their output voltage must be amplified in the device before they can be modified to produce the desired pulses

The DC voltage is now transformed into trains of pulses by one or more oscillators. Pulse shape, pulse repetition rate, number and distribution of pulses within a pulse train, etc., are determined in the oscillator stage of the stimulator (Cook 1987). The final stage of the unit amplifies the desired waveform to the required amplitude for a given therapeutic procedure. The amplification and hence the signal amplitude, can be controlled by the operator by means of a control dial on the TENS device. Unfortunately, the divisions marked on the device around the dial are generally not calibrated in terms of volts or amperes, but are in arbitrary units from 0 to 10. As already illustrated in Figure 3.13, these scales are not, as one would expect, linear. Indeed Campbell (1982) has shown in a range of TENS models that increasing the amplification 'slightly' at the upper end of the scale may in fact lead to a disproportionately large increase in the applied current or voltage, with obvious risk to the patient (Fig. 4.2).

Campbell also reported similar findings for the dials which control pulse frequency (Fig. 4.3).

In general, TENS units have two channels for independent stimulation and each channel of signal amplitude can be independently controlled. The output current or voltage from a TENS device should, theoretically, be constant once set and should not vary with time or from patient to patient. Campbell (1982) found that many units have current outputs which change as the interelectrode impedance (or 'load') varies (Fig. 4.4). It was observed that as a load was decreased, the applied current in some devices increased dramatically. As there are interhuman variations in skin impedance, at best the above observation means that with these devices, comparisons between patients are meaningless. At worst, it is downright dangerous, since a given patient's skin impedance will probably decrease during therapy, resulting in an unexpected increase in the amplitude of the applied current.

It is therefore not altogether surprising that Campbell (1982) concluded that many TENS devices 'are not so sophisticated as perhaps the manufacturers' literature (and some of their

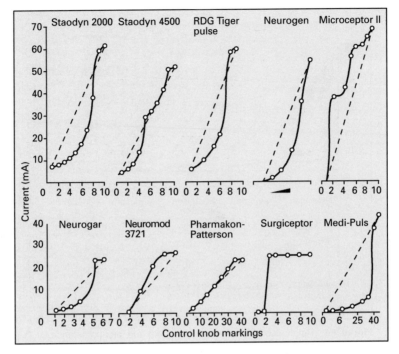

Figure 4.2 TENS amplitude control calibration curves with a 1 kΩ load. Dashed lines denote curves for linear calibration. (From Campbell 1982, with permission.)

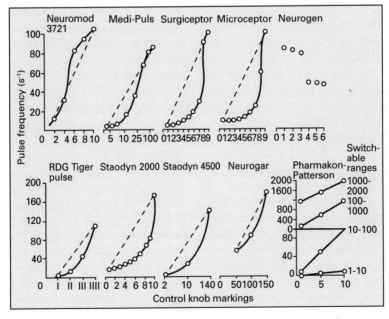

Figure 4.3 TENS frequency control dial calibration curves. Dashed lines denote curves for linear calibration. The Neurogen* had six switchable positions which simultaneously changed frequency and pulse duration. (From Campbell 1982, with permission.)

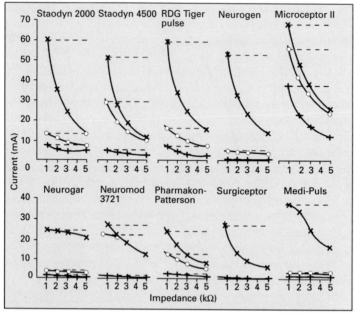

Figure 4.4 Relationship between output current and load impedance for low (+), mid-range (o) and high (x) settings of the amplitude control dial. Dashed line denotes curves for constant current output. (From Campbell 1982, with permission.)

prices) would have us believe'. It is difficult to carry out meaningful research into the effects of various parameters such as pulse amplitude, frequency, etc., and to use the conclusions so drawn in effective therapy if the devices one is using are of such quality. AC-powered units are probably better than small 'low cost', light-weight, battery-powered units in this regard (Cook 1987).

Constant current or constant voltage

Most TENS units are designed with either constant current or constant voltage output, the former being the most common as it is the level of the current and not the voltage which is responsible for causing the desired physiological effects. Theoretically, the delivered current or voltage amplitude will remain constant irrespective of any changes in impedance of the electrode/patient system.

With a constant voltage unit, the delivered current will depend on the electrode–patient imped-ance and the current will vary from patient to patient, from site to site and from one electrode system to another. A decrease in an electrode's impedance with time, due, for example, to applied pressure, will cause the current intensity to increase with the risk of causing pain to the patient. On the other hand, for example, if an electrode starts to peel off the skin causing the contact impedance to increase, the constant voltage unit will automatically compensate and decrease the current flowing through the reduced contact area, thus decreasing the risk of burns to the patient due to localised high current densities. Due to the capacitive nature of the electrode–patient impedance, a relatively large current will flow at the start of the pulse and the current amplitude will then decrease during the pulse duration. Although the initial peak in current may be of a sufficient amplitude to elicit the desired response, the effective duration of the pulse may be a lot less than the duration of the applied voltage pulse.

A constant current unit will theoretically maintain the same current regardless of changes in loading impedance. As it is the level of current and not the voltage which is responsible for causing the desired physiological effect, it is more logical to control the applied current. This enables more meaningful therapy and research. If, however, the electrode gradually peels off or if the contact area decreases for any other reason, the current density in the remaining area will increase, with the risk of causing pain and burns to the patient. According to Ohm's law (V = IR), in order for the same current (I) to flow through a smaller contact area with its larger impedance (R), the driving voltage (V) of the system must increase. Well-designed constant current units therefore incorporate circuitry which limits the device's maximum voltage output in order to minimise or eliminate the risk of passing excessive current densities through the patient.

THE ELECTRICAL PROPERTIES OF THE ELECTRODE–SKIN INTERFACE

The electrode–gel–skin interface

In order to apply effective therapeutic electrical impulses to a patient, a suitable stimulator must be connected electrically (via flexible insulated wires called electrode leads or cables) to at least one pair of electrodes attached to the patient's skin at locations judged by the therapist to be optimal for achieving the desired effect.

A basic TENS electrode system appears relatively simple and generally comprises a conductive disc or plate, an ion-containing gel, a means of attachment to the skin and a means of connection to the stimulator's lead. However, of all the component parts of the overall TENS system, the electrode–gel–skin interface has probably been the least understood and the most problematic (Mannheimer & Lampe 1984). Quite apart from influencing the effectiveness of the treatment, poor electrode design can give rise to electrically-, chemically- and mechanically-induced skin irritation and trauma to the patient.

One of the functions of the electrodes is to ensure good electrical contact between the patient's skin and the stimulator's leads. The electrodes must, therefore, at the very least, make firm mechanical contact with the skin. As the current or charge delivered by the stimulator is carried by electrons in the device itself and in its leads, and by ions inside the patient's body, there must be a change in current/charge carrier at the electrode–patient interface. The 'charge transfer' mechanism which occurs at the electrode–body interface is therefore of major importance in the design of an optimal electrode device. One must not simply choose an electrode with as conductive a metal or carbon-loaded plate as possible.

The electrode device must not only ensure good electrical contact between the stimulator and the patient and facilitate the transfer of charge across the electrode–body interface, but it must also help to decrease the large electrical impedance of the dry, dead outer layers of the patient's skin if effective, trauma-free stimulation is to be achieved.

The distribution of current density under an electrode is another important parameter. If, for whatever reason, a large portion of the applied current flows into the patient through only a small area of the electrode–skin interface, high current density 'hot spots' can occur and considerable pain and trauma can be caused to the patient when applying apparently 'safe' therapeutic impulses.

Electrode technology is therefore important to the effective, atraumatic use of TENS and is not as simple as it might first appear. The design of the electrodes, the materials used in their construction, the electrode sizes and shapes, the method of attachment, all need to be carefully considered when choosing an optimal electrode for a given application.

The electrode–gel interface

Interesting and rather complex things occur when an electrode is placed in contact with an electrolyte gel (or body fluids such as sweat). It has already been stated that in the electrode and the connecting lead, electrical charge is carried by electrons whereas in the gel and body, charge is carried by ions. There is a transition at the interface between the electrode and the electrolyte

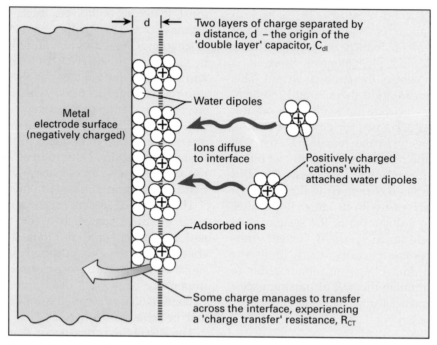

Figure 4.5 Schematic representation of the electrode–gel interface.

where the charge is transferred from one kind of carrier to the other (McAdams et al 1995). The charges which transfer across the interface can experience a significant 'charge transfer' resistance, R_{CT} (Fig. 4.5).

In order for some of the ions in the electrode gel or in the body fluids to transfer their charge across the interface, many must first diffuse to the interface. Here they 'stick' (or 'adsorb' as it is termed in electrochemistry) to the electrode surface. If the electrode has a negative charge relative to the electrolyte, positive ions will be attracted to the interface region and will 'stick' to the electrode surface. As a consequence, there is a layer of charge on the metal surface and a layer of equal but opposite charge on the electrolyte side of the interface, both separated by a small distance. A 'double layer' of charge therefore exists at the interface and such a system behaves like a parallel plate capacitor (a capacitor is a device which can store quantities of electrical charge; capacitance is the ability of a capacitor to store charge). Not altogether surprisingly, the interface's capacitance is often termed the double layer capacitance, C_{dl}, and is connected in parallel

to the charge transfer resistance (R_{CT}) in our simple equivalent circuit model (Fig. 4.6).

In order to understand some aspects of the double layer capacitance, it is helpful to consider the basic equation for a parallel plate capacitor. If two identical conductive plates, each of area A cm^2 are separated by a distance d cm which is filled with a material of dielectric constant k (Fig. 4.7), then the capacitance of this parallel plate capacitor, C_{pp}, is given by:

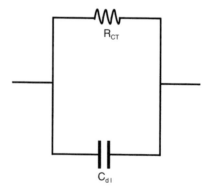

Figure 4.6 Equivalent circuit model of the electrode–gel interface.

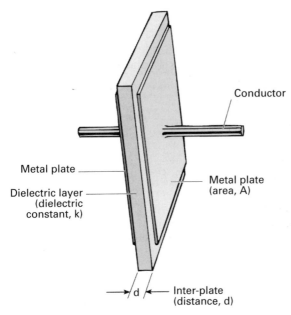

Conductor

Metal plate

Dielectric layer
(dielectric
constant, k)

Metal plate
(area, A)

d

Inter-plate
(distance, d)

Figure 4.7 Parallel plate capacitor.

$$C_{pp} = 0.0885\ \frac{Ak}{d} \qquad \text{(Equation 1)}$$

The magnitude of the parallel plate capacitive impedance, Z_{pp}, is given by:

$$Z_{pp} = \frac{1}{2\pi f C_{pp}} \qquad \text{(Equation 2)}$$

where f is the frequency of the applied AC signal and π is a constant. (*Note*: Impedance is a more general concept than resistance as it takes into account the additional effects of capacitance.)

An electron which is forced into one 'plate' of the capacitor will not be able to travel through the dielectric, non-conducting material to the other plate. Due to the thinness of the dielectric material, the electrical field of the electron can, however, propagate through the dielectric and repels an electron away from the second plate (Cromwell et al 1976), making the latter positively charged; the electron therefore appears to pass through the capacitor. The electron on the first plate and the positive charge on the second plate attract each other and hold each other in place. A capacitor therefore has the ability to store electrical charges and hence to store energy. The energy stored in a capacitor is a consequence

of the electrical fields generated by the many mutually attracting charges at the plates. The larger the capacitor plates or the thinner the dielectric layer, the larger the number of charges which can be stored and the larger the capacitor's 'capacity' (see Equation 1). Although a direct current cannot flow through a capacitor, the interaction of voltages on either side of the dielectric enables the 'apparent' flow of alternating current. As the amplitude and direction of an alternating current change with time, the changing field at the first plate produces a changing field at the second plate. Although electrons do not in fact flow through the capacitor, alternating current (or any time varying current) is passed across the capacitor. The more rapidly an applied signal varies with time, the more readily it passes through a capacitor.

The electrical impedance of a capacitor is therefore inversely proportional to the frequency of the applied AC signal as described in Equation 2. If a very high frequency AC signal is applied to a capacitor, the impedance of the capacitor diminishes towards zero and current flows through the capacitor practically unopposed. If the applied signal's frequency is zero, i.e. if a DC signal is applied, the capacitor's impedance tends to infinity and direct current can not flow through it. The effect of TENS pulses rather than AC is considered in detail in Appendix I.

Polarisation

As direct current cannot flow through the capacitance C_{dl} in the equivalent circuit, all of an applied direct current, i_{dc}, must flow through the resistance R_{CT} which is in parallel with C_{dl} (Fig. 4.6). The voltage dropped across this charge transfer resistance will be equal to i_{dc} multiplied by R_{CT} (from Ohm's law: V = IR). This change in the electrode interface's potential from its equilibrium value (measured in the absence of an applied direct current) is termed 'polarisation'. An electrode system with a very large value of charge transfer resistance will develop a large additional voltage (or 'over-potential' as it is termed in electrochemistry) due to the presence of R_{CT}, and the electrode is said to be highly polarisable. An electrode system which has a very low value of R_{CT} lets current traverse the interface almost unimpeded, there is little energy wasted at the interface, the over-potential is relatively small and the electrode system is relatively non-polarisable (McAdams et al 1995). Such electrode systems, which let current flow through them almost unimpeded, are highly sought after, especially when recording small biosignals.

Electrode materials

A good electrode material must have good conductivity, must give rise to low interface impedances (including low polarisation, i.e. R_{CT}) and must not produce irritating or toxic by-products when used on patients.

Silver-silver chloride electrodes, when used in conjunction with chloride-containing gels, have relatively high values of C_{dl} and low values of R_{CT}. As a consequence they are often used in ECG electrodes. A silver-silver chloride electrode plate is made by electrolytically coating a piece of pure silver with silver chloride. The resulting silver chloride layer facilitates the transfer of charge between the silver metal and the chloride-based electrolyte and this electrode system is characterised by a small value of charge transfer resistance (McAdams et al 1992).

Early workers in TENS used silver-silver chloride and other electrodes originally intended for biosignal monitoring. Such electrodes could not, however, cope with the relatively long term application of large current levels. In the case of a silver-silver chloride electrode, the silver chloride layer was either (depending on the polarity of the electrode):

- quickly removed, or
- became too thick and effectively blocked the electrode surface with a resistive coating (silver chloride is highly resistive).

Silver-silver chloride electrodes are still used (very rarely) for some short term TENS applications.

The majority of commercially available TENS electrodes are now moulded from an elastomer such as silicone rubber or a plastic such as ethyl-ene vinyl acetate and loaded with electrically conductive carbon black (finely divided carbon particles). Such electrodes can be moulded into almost any size or shape and they are relatively very flexible, making them suitable for a wide range of both short term and long term TENS applications. More recently, many reusable and disposable electrodes based on thin conductive foils, meshes or clothes have become popular.

Compared to silver-silver chloride, all of the above materials are highly polarisable (i.e. have larger values of R_{CT}) and tend to have smaller values of double layer capacitance (i.e. higher values of high frequency capacitive impedance). It must be pointed out that the electrode–gel interface impedance (due to the parallel combination of R_{CT} and C_{dl}) is relatively unimportant compared to the large skin impedance and although the above shortcomings would be considered important in biosignal monitoring, they are less so in TENS.

Mannheimer & Lampe (1984) have pointed out that the only tangible disadvantage of having a large electrode impedance is that more power will be required from the stimulator to drive the stimulating current through the electrodes into the body and achieve the desired stimulation. As a consequence, there may be some reduction in battery life.

THE SKIN
Structure of the skin

The skin is a multilayered organ which covers and protects the body. The skin has several functions and its structure is well adapted for these tasks. Due to its poor thermal conductivity, it provides an effective protection against variations in temperature. As it is solid, elastic and self-repairing, the skin protects the body against everyday 'wear and tear'. The structure of the skin makes it an extremely efficient barrier, capable of keeping water within the body and unwanted foreign compounds and parasites out of the body. The presence of numerous sensory nerve endings in the skin enables sensations of touch, pressure, pain and temperature. The skin produces two secretions: the secretion of the sebaceous glands keeps the skin smooth and waterproof while sweat, through its evaporation, enables the body to lose heat and helps excrete some waste products.

The skin is made up of three principal layers – the subcutaneous layer, the dermis and the epidermis (Fig. 4.8). (*Note*: In the literature, the terminology used to denote these layers varies.) The subcutaneous layer is a layer of connective tissue and is one of the body's areas for storing fat. This layer enables the skin on most parts of the body to move freely over underlying structures. The dermis constitutes the greater part of the skin proper (approximately 2 mm thick) and is formed of a dense network of connective tissue. It contains numerous blood vessels, hair follicles, sebaceous and sweat glands and several types of sensory nerve endings.

The epidermis can be around 100 μm thick, depending on body site. The epidermis can be further subdivided into several layers with the 'basal layer' forming the innermost layer and the stratum corneum the outermost layer. Cells in the basal layer are constantly multiplying and as they are pushed up towards the skin's external surface, the cells undergo changes. From their initial cubical form they gradually become flattened, compacted, dehydrated, lose their nuclei and develop a hardening protein (keratin). Eventually, such cells (called corneocytes) form the stratum corneum which has a thickness of around 15 μm, depending on its hydration and body location. These dead cells are continuously being shed with constant replacement from the underlying epidermal layers.

The epidermal layer is traversed by numerous skin appendages such as hair follicles, sebaceous glands and sweat glands. The average skin surface is believed to contain 40–70 hair follicles and 200–250 sweat ducts per square centimetre.

Electrical properties of the skin

The impedance of the skin is the largest component of the overall interelectrode impedance (Fig. 4.9). When a dry (i.e. non-gelled) conductive electrode is placed on the skin of a patient, the dead stratum corneum layer presents a very high impedance to the transmission of an applied direct current since ions have difficulty in traversing this dry barrier. If the stratum corneum was as hydrated with conductive body fluids as the underlying tissues, current would flow through with little problem.

Although the stratum corneum will not let much direct current flow through it, due to its thinness and its dielectric properties, it will allow the interaction of electrical potentials across it. One can imagine the relatively non-conductive stratum corneum sandwiched between the con-

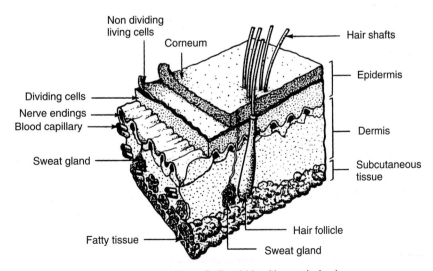

Figure 4.8 Structure of the skin. (From Reilly 1992, with permission.)

ductive electrode and the conductive tissues underlying the stratum corneum. This has the makings of a parallel plate capacitor where two conductive plates are separated by a non-conducting dielectric material (see Equation 1). The stratum corneum's electrical impedance is therefore often represented by a simple capacitor, C_{SP} (Fig. 4.9).

Some ions do manage to cross the stratum corneum barrier and this flow of current is represented by a large resistance, R_{SP}, in parallel with the above capacitance. It must be borne in mind that this equivalent circuit model is a simplification of the rather complex electrical properties of the skin. It will, however, be sufficient for this present discussion. The skin's parallel capacitance dominates its electrical behaviour at high frequencies as its impedance is much smaller than R_{SP} in this frequency range (above a few kHz). R_{SP} dominates the skin's low frequency behaviour (below 1 Hz). In Appendix I, it is shown that C_{SP} dominates the skin's initial electrical response to an applied step or pulse of voltage or current while R_{SP} dominates the response for longer durations.

The skin's parallel capacitance (C_{SP})

It was suggested above that the electrode–skin interface can be approximated by a capacitor with the stratum corneum forming the dielectric layer sandwiched between the electrode and the underlying tissues which form the conductive plates. It can be seen from Equation 1 that the skin's capacitance will increase (its capacitive impedance, Z_{SP}, will decrease – Equation 2) as the area of the electrode increases, the thickness of the stratum corneum decreases or its dielectric constant increases.

As the thickness and composition of the stratum corneum can vary over the body, or from patient to patient, variations have been observed in skin capacitance (for a given electrode area). The capacitance of the skin is typically within the range 0.02–$0.06\ \mu F/cm^2$ when measured using electrodes with 'wet' electrolyte gels several minutes after electrode application (Yamamoto & Yamamoto 1978). Given that the surface of the skin is irregular, a flat dry electrode will only make contact with a few 'peaks' on the skin surface and hence there is a smaller effective contact

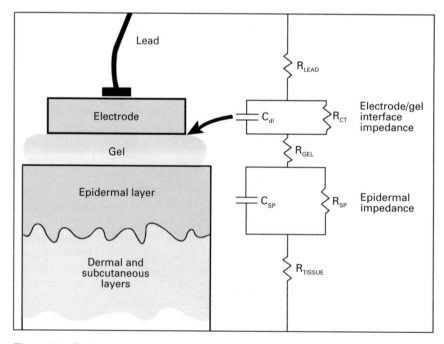

Figure 4.9 Equivalent circuit model of the electrode–gel–skin interface.

area than expected. This will give rise to smaller values of C_{SP} than cited above. However, as sweat builds up under the occlusive, dry electrodes, a better contact with the skin will result in a gradual increase in the measured value of C_{SP}. A similar, though much more rapid, effect is observed when a 'wet' gelled electrode is initially placed on the skin and the gel spreads over the skin and into the pores and crevices (McAdams & Jossinet 1991).

The skin's parallel resistance (R_{SP})

Although the stratum corneum does not easily allow foreign substances to traverse it, some current, carried by ions, manages to flow through it. The difficulty or resistance this current experiences in passing through the skin is represented in our equivalent circuit by the parallel resistance, R_{SP}. This ionic current is believed to flow through:

• the skin appendages, which act as shunts through the stratum corneum to the interior, and
• via paracellular (around cells) pathways.

The dominant pathway appears to depend on the applied signal amplitude. Although the skin's appendages (sweat glands, etc.) occupy only approximately 0.1% of the skin's surface, large currents appear to seek out these paths of least resistance and a significant portion of such currents can flow through the skin's appendages. In any case, the skin's resistance is highly dependent on the presence and activity of sweat glands and on the presence of other appendageal pathways. R_{SP} varies greatly from patient to patient, from body site to body site and with time. The density of sweat glands varies from approximately 370 per cm^2 on the palms of the hands and the soles of the feet to approximately 160 per cm^2 on the forearm (Reilly 1992). The measured values of R_{SP} are much smaller on areas with high densities of sweat glands, such as the palms of the hands (in spite of the thicker stratum corneum layer), especially when the glands are active in response to thermal or psychophysiological stimuli (McAdams & Jossinet 1991).

Electrode gels and their effects

Electrode gels serve:

• to ensure a good electrical contact between the electrode and the patient's skin
• to facilitate the transfer of charge at the electrode–gel interface between the two kinds of charge carrier (electrons in the electrode and ions in the gel)
• to decrease the large impedance of the stratum corneum.

There are two main types of electrode gel – aqueous, 'wet' gels (often termed gels, pastes, creams or jellies) and hydrogels.

'Wet' gels. 'Wet' gels are generally made of water, a thickening agent, a bactericide/fungicide and an ionic salt (Carim 1988). When the gel is applied to the skin it rapidly fills up the 'troughs' on the electrode and skin surfaces, thus ensuring maximum effective contact area. The ions in the gel serve not only to ensure electrical conductivity of the gel but also to decrease the skin impedance by diffusing into the skin due to the existing concentration gradient.

The impedance of the gel layer can be represented by a simple resistance in series with the impedances of the skin and the electrode–gel interface. The magnitude of the gel resistance will depend on the composition and concentration of the gel and on the dimensions of the gel layer. Tissue fluids and sweat largely contain sodium, potassium and chloride ions. In order to ensure biocompatibility, the ionic salts most commonly used in electrode gels for biosignal monitoring are NaCl (sodium chloride) and KCl (potassium chloride). High concentrations of these salts tend to be better tolerated by the body than other salts. Higher salt concentrations give rise to a more rapid diffusion of ions into the skin and a more rapid decrease in the skin's parallel resistance (R_{SP}). The skin's capacitance (C_{SP}) tends to increase with increasing salt concentration. However, even with sodium chloride, the concentration of the salt cannot be increased indefinitely as it will eventually give rise to skin irritation problems.

In the previous paragraph it has been stated

that, for electrode gels used in biosignal recording applications, one must be careful not to use too high a concentration of electrolyte salt in order to avoid skin trauma. This problem is even more important in TENS as the applied large-amplitude impulses actively 'push' large amounts of the irritating ions electrophoretically into the patient's skin.

As pointed out previously, although a low skin impedance is desirable, it is not as critical in TENS as it is in biosignal monitoring. Electrode gels with high concentrations of electrolyte, with their increased skin irritation potential, are not therefore used in TENS. In fact, non-chloride based electrolytes are generally used in order to minimise skin irritation problems (Carim 1988).

Hydrogels. Hydrogels are the second kind of electrode gel commonly used in TENS electrode systems. Hydrogels are 'solid' gels which incorporate natural (e.g. karaya gum, a polysaccharide obtained from a tree found in India) or synthetic (e.g. polyvinyl pyrrolidone) hydrocolloids (Carim 1988). Hydrogels tend to be more resistive than 'wet' gels. The highest resistivity hydrogels tend to be used in stimulating electrodes (see below) and the lowest resistivity 'wet' gels used for biosignal monitoring.

Hydrogels accommodate the contours and irregularities of the surfaces of the skin and the electrode and hence increase the effective contact area between the electrode and the skin compared to dry electrode systems. However, being hydrophilic (i.e. they absorb water), they are poor at hydrating the skin and may even absorb the skin's surface moisture. They are therefore not only more resistive than 'wet' gels, but they hydrate the skin less effectively and give rise to higher skin impedances (i.e. higher values of R_{SP} and lower values of C_{SP}) (McAdams & Jossinet 1991). As previously pointed out, this increase is not necessarily a significant disadvantage in TENS applications and, as will be shown, may even be an advantage.

A further advantage of using hydrogels is that they cause less skin irritation compared to 'wet' gels. A simplistic explanation of the advantageous/disadvantageous features of hydrogels is that hydrogels serve principally to ensure a good electrical contact between the skin and the electrode and that they do not significantly affect (compared to 'wet' gels) the properties of the stratum corneum, either to improve or degrade.

The electrical properties of the gel layer can be represented by a simple resistor (R_{GEL}), as shown in Figure 4.9.

Electrode and skin preparation

Arguably the most important aspect of the electrode–skin interface in TENS is the quality of contact between the electrode and the skin. One must strive to ensure that, as far as possible, the current flowing through the patient's skin is distributed as evenly as possible across the whole of the interface. The entire surfaces of the electrode and the skin must participate in the transfer of charge. No portion of the surfaces should be blocked by an insulating layer and the gel must penetrate deep into surface 'troughs' and pores.

Reusable electrodes (such as carbon-loaded silicone) must be cleaned with a mild soap solution after every application to avoid the formation and build-up of blocking layers of residue on the electrode surface. The skin's surface can also be washed to remove some of the loose, outermost cells of the stratum corneum and this also tends to degrease the skin's surface. This technique has the added advantage of 'pre-wetting' the skin before electrode application.

Care must be taken when degreasing the skin with alcohol as it may initially increase the impedance of the skin by further dehydrating the outermost layers of the skin. However, in the case of 'wet' gelled electrodes, the gel does penetrate more rapidly into skin. This may not be the case with hydrogel-based electrodes.

The outer layers of the stratum corneum can be removed by rubbing the skin with abrasive pads especially designed for this purpose. This can give rise to a major decrease in R_{SP} and an increase in C_{SP} (McAdams & Jossinet 1991). Skin 'stripping' is a technique where the stratum corneum is progressively removed, using adhesive tape which is repeatedly placed on the skin and then pulled off. However, great care must be taken, especially in TENS applications, to avoid causing skin irritation due to the use of a high concentration gel or to the use of abrasion techniques.

Overall impedance

A simple equivalent circuit model for the electrode–gel–skin system is shown in Figure 4.10. This has been simplified by assuming that the skin impedance is much higher than the electrode–gel interface impedance and by ignoring the latter. One is therefore left with the impedance of the skin site in series with the resistances of the gel layers and the underlying tissues.

However, two electrodes are used to apply the TENS impulses and the contributions of both electrode–gel–skin interfaces ought to be taken into account. Skin (and the electrode–gel interface) impedance is inversely proportioned to the gelled area. If one of the two electrodes used to apply a therapeutic impulse is very small compared to the second (e.g. when the smaller of the two is being used to apply accurately an impulse to a small target area such as a motor point), the impedance of the larger electrode is much smaller and is often ignored, leaving the equivalent circuit shown on Figure 4.10. R_S represents the sum of the series resistances due to the leads, gel pads and the underlying tissues.

If both electrodes have the same surface area, then it is often assumed (erroneously) that they have identical impedances. Both skin impedances can then be combined to give an equivalent circuit similar to that shown on Figure 4.10. In both of the above cases, one is left with a simple (emphasis on the word 'simple'), '3-component' equivalent circuit model of the electrical properties of the total electrode/patient system.

If very low frequency AC (e.g. less than 1 Hz) or a direct current is applied to the above equivalent circuit model, most/all of the current will flow through the resistances R_{SP} and R_S as the capacitor C_{SP} presents a very large impedance to low frequency signals (see Equation 2). The total impedance at low frequencies is therefore large, purely resistive and equal to:

$$Z_{\text{Low frequency}} = R_{SP} + R_S \qquad \text{(Equation 3)}$$

At very high frequencies (more than 1 kHz), the current tends to flow through the capacitor unhindered and, as R_{SP} is effectively bypassed, the current only encounters the resistance R_S. Once again, the impedance is purely resistive, though in this case, relatively, very small, with a resistance value equal to the sum of the lead, electrode (not interface), gel and underlying tissue resistance:

$$Z_{\text{High frequency}} = R_S \qquad \text{(Equation 4)}$$

As the magnitude of the capacitor's impedance decreases with the frequency of the applied AC current or voltage, at intermediate frequencies the capacitor lets some current through it and the total impedance to the flow of current decreases. This behaviour can be clearly seen in Figure 4.11 which is a plot of the logarithm of the magnitude of the impedance versus the logarithm of the frequency of the applied AC signal.

Importance of electrode–skin impedance

In TENS, one is using surface electrodes to deliver energy to targeted nerves, whether they are located in the skin or in underlying tissues. Tissues have differing resistive and capacitive properties. When a given impulse is applied to a patient, the amount of energy which 'reaches' a given tissue depends on its relative electrical resistance compared to those of other tissues in the electrical field. (Variations in current density

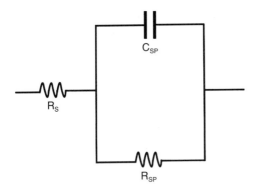

Figure 4.10   Simple '3-component' model of the inter-electrode impedance.

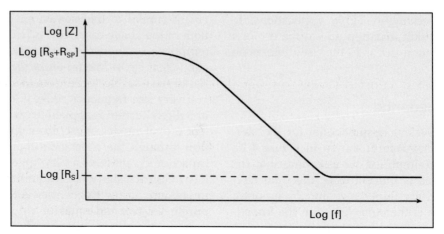

Figure 4.11 Bode plot (log of the impedance magnitude versus log of frequency) for the impedance of the '3-component' model.

have been ignored in this simple explanation. It is assumed that tissues form layers, one on top of another.) As energy consumed by a resistance is equal to I^2R, a high resistance tissue, such as the skin, will 'consume' more of the available energy (which, in this case is converted to heat) and leave relatively little for a neighbouring low resistance tissue. Not only does this cause local irritation and vasodilation in the skin, but is somewhat unfortunate if the nerves one hopes to stimulate are located in an underlying tissue with low electrical resistance. The problem is further complicated by the frequency dependence of some of the tissues' impedances (or effective resistances). The skin is an important example.

For direct current and for slowly changing pulses of current, the skin's capacitive impedance is very large and hence the skin's effective resistance is very high relative to the resistance of the underlying tissues. Most of the applied energy is therefore 'used up' by the skin and subcutaneous tissues and it is cutaneous nerves which are principally affected (Low & Reed 1994). For short, high frequency pulses of current, the skin's impedance is less significant and a higher portion of the energy is dissipated in the deeper tissues.

Short duration pulses (around 0.05 ms) should therefore be more able to 'penetrate through the skin and into the deeper tissues and this should

be more efficient at stimulating low threshold nerves which are located below the skin. It has also been suggested that high threshold unmyelinated nociceptive fibres (C fibres) located in the skin should be more effectively stimulated using longer pulses (Low & Reed 1994).

Current density

In the simplest case, current density (the amount of current per unit of conduction area) is inversely proportional to the electrode/skin contact area. If the same current is applied through a pair of large electrodes and a pair of small electrodes, the stimulation effect will be most pronounced under the small area electrodes due to the increased current density. If a small electrode is used in conjunction with a large area electrode, the effect is more pronounced under the smaller of the two. In this case, the small electrode is often used as the 'active' electrode to target a small area such as a motor point. The large electrode is simply used to complete the electrical circuit and is termed the 'indifferent' or 'dispersive' electrode.

Under a given electrode, it is highly desirable to have a uniform current density, as the increased concentration of the current at one or more points under the electrode may cause pain and trauma to the patient at otherwise safe overall current densities. At best in such cases, the applied current may have to be limited to less than therapeutic values due to the patient's discomfort (Carim 1988).

With the old-fashioned rigid metal plate electrodes which were strapped to the body, current density 'hot spots' could occur if all of the electrode, due to the contours of the body, did not make good electrical contact with the skin.

Wrinkles in malleable metal electrodes can encourage preferential current flow through small areas of the gel and into the patient. Even with the commonly used carbon rubber electrodes, 'wet' gels can squeeze out from under parts of the electrode and give rise to increased current densities in other areas. The use of hydrogel minimises this problem source (Carim 1988).

With highly conductive metal electrodes, such as those used for external cardiac pacing, defibrillation or electrosurgery, current density hot spots occur under the perimeter of the electrode. The current density at the perimeter can be around three times higher than that at the centre of the electrode (Caruso et al 1979). Although calculating or measuring the current density distribution profile under an electrode can be difficult, a simple intuitive picture will aid the understanding of many of the main features.

When current flows into a highly conductive metal electrode, it has the choice of continuing to flow through the conductive metal or into the more resistive gel–skin interface. Like most of us, the electrical current chooses the path of least resistance and much of it continues to flow through the metal until it reaches the perimeter of the plate where it then is forced to flow through the gel into the patient. It should be remembered that if the two electrodes used to apply an impulse are placed too close together, the current tends to flow through the shortest path and hence tends to flow through the edge closest to the neighbouring electrode rather than through the whole of the electrode–skin interface.

In TENS, relatively resistive conductive rubber is used and the opposite problem arises. When current is introduced into the conductive rubber (via a small metallic connector), it prefers to flow

into the skin immediately under the connector rather than laterally through the resistive electrode. Efforts to overcome this problem include incorporating conductive elements in the rubber to help spread the current more evenly over the entire interface surface (Fig. 4.12). Some electrodes have a thin metallic layer coated onto the back of the conductive rubber and these appear to give rise to the most uniform current density profiles (Carim 1988).

The electrical properties of carbon rubber electrodes deteriorate with time. Areas of the electrode will no longer conduct properly, leading to increases in current density at certain points and to the increased possibility of causing pain to the patient. 'Reusable' carbon rubber electrodes should therefore be replaced every 3–6 months.

Skin irritation

Skin irritation problems can arise from a wide range of possible sources, e.g. mechanical, chemical and thermal.

The relative shearing of skin's dermal and epidermal layers can give rise to mechanically-induced irritation. This can result from the way in which an electrode's adhesive tape is applied to the skin or to subsequent movement or deformation of the electrode relative to the underlying tissues. For example, if long strips of tape or long electrodes are attached to the skin in parallel with the patient's spinal column, the act of bending forward on the part of the patient will produce very strong shearing stresses within the skin (Mannheimer & Lampe 1984). Such possibilities should be taken into account when applying electrodes, especially those incorporating or requiring adhesive tapes. The problem will be most marked for certain relatively inelastic foam and 'paper' tapes. Soft, stretchable cloth-like materials should help minimise the problems as they tend to accommodate, to some extent at least, skin movement and deformation. Adhesive hydrogel-based electrodes (thus not requiring adhesive tapes) also tend to be good in this respect.

In the past, electrodes containing rigid gel-retaining rings (such as one finds in the standard ECG electrode) had the potential of causing

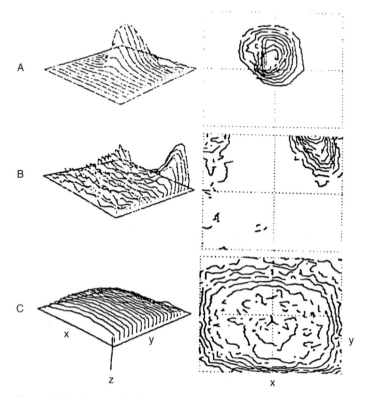

Figure 4.12 Current distribution profiles of stimulating electrodes. Left: Profile of z-axis component of surface current vector. Right: Equal current contour lines in x–y plane for the corresponding electrode on the left. (A) ECG electrode with gel and snap connector. (B) Carbon–silicone rubber electrode patch with gel. (C) Metal–vapor-coated carbon rubber CA (conductive adhesive) electrode. Plots derived using 4 mA current pulses from TENS stimulator. (From Carim 1988. Reprinted by permission of John Wiley & Sons, Inc.)

mechanically-induced irritation due to the rings pressing and rubbing against the skin – for example, when worn by a bedridden patient or attached under a patient during a surgical procedure. Electrode connectors and leads can also cause similar problems. Mechanically-induced skin irritation can also result from skin stripping during tape removal. This problem is more pronounced when the skin layers are moist due, for example, to the use of an occlusive tape.

If the skin surface is occluded, sweat builds up under the impermeable barrier and the warm, moist conditions are ideal for bacterial growth. Impermeable, adhesive, foam tapes are especially susceptible to this problem. Porous backing tapes allow the skin to breathe and lose moisture,

thus minimising the problem. Hydrogels tend to absorb skin surface moisture and are generally characterised by low incidences of skin irritation problems.

It is difficult (or impossible) to find a material which can be worn on the skin by all patients without causing some form of allergic reaction in at least some of the patients. The adhesives now coated onto backing tapes tend to be hypoallergenic acrylate adhesives which, because they allow water vapour transmission, are non-occlusive (Carim 1988). Porous backing tapes tend to cause the least number of problems as, amongst other things, the area of adhesive coverage is reduced and often the adhesives used are milder.

Irritation can arise as a result of the composition and concentration of the electrode gel. Unlike biosignal monitoring electrode gels, high concentration electrode gels, with their increased skin irritation potential, are not used in TENS. TENS gels incorporate a non-chloride ion salt and typically use glycerine instead of propylene glycol due to the increased skin irritation potential which exists with the high currents used in TENS (Carim 1988). Some gels, often for biosignal monitoring, include chemical or abrasive irritants to reduce the electrical impedance of the skin. These should be avoided for TENS. Hydrogels such as karaya tend not to actively interact with the skin and are relatively hypoallergenic.

Nickel, which may be a component of the snap fasteners used in some electrode designs, may cause reactions in sensitive patients. TENS electrodes are now generally made of conductive rubber in order to avoid corrosion products from metal electrodes causing skin irritations. Very few irritation or allergic skin reactions have been reported for conductive rubber electrodes (Mannheimer & Lampe 1984).

High current densities can cause tissue injury due to, among other things, heating effects. It has been stated that the heat produced beneath an electrode must be less than $250 \, mcal/cm^2/sec^3$ and that, as a consequence, the electrode surface area of a TENS electrode must be equal to or greater than $4 \, cm^2$ skin (Mannheimer & Lampe 1984). High current density 'hot spots' can, however, still occur due to faulty electrode design, electrode ageing, poor electrode application, improper gelling of the electrode, etc.

If one were to apply direct current (DC) through the electrode–skin interface, the by-products of the electrochemical reactions involved in the charge transfer process would diffuse into the skin, causing chemical injury to the skin. When one is applying pulses of current to a patient, the current initially flows into the patient via the electrode–gel capacitance (Appendix I, Fig. 4.9). Generally, as there is no reaction associated with the capacitive flow of current, there are few undesirable effects when using very short duration pulses. As the pulse duration is increased, progressively more current flows through the parallel resistance. This is characterised by a 'levelling off' of the voltage response as it tends towards its limiting value of $V\infty$ (Appendix I, Fig. A1). Current flows through the parallel resistance as a result of electrochemical reactions and hence such current flow is more likely to give rise to skin irritation. Long duration pulses should therefore be avoided. Modern TENS systems generate pulses with very short pulse durations, of the order of 100 or 200 microseconds.

When a TENS current is applied in one direction through the electrode–patient interface, some of the by-products of the electrochemical reactions involved may diffuse into the patient's skin and give rise to irritation. In the past, in electrotherapy, electrodes were used with thick pads of electrolyte-impregnated lint in order to distance the patient's skin from the electrode–electrolyte interface and the undesirable by-products. In using 'charge balanced' waveforms in modern TENS devices, it is often believed that because there is no net charge transfer across the electrode–skin interface, there is also no net flow of potentially harmful by-products into the skin (see section on zero net DC in Ch. 3). What is produced in one phase is thought to be 'recaptured' in the second. Unfortunately, the electrochemical reaction which occurs to enable the flow of current during the first phase is not necessarily that involved in the second. By-products of the first reaction are therefore not always 'recaptured' and may 'escape' from the interface and reach the patient. However, it must be pointed out that the use of charge-balanced biphasic waveforms does indeed greatly minimise the problem; hence its widespread use.

TENS ELECTRODES
Electrode size and shape

Initially, electrodes originally designed for ECG and other biosignal monitoring applications were used with TENS units. Some still are. Larger, more suitable electrode designs were eventually developed in order to reduce the current densities under the electrodes, to reduce skin irritation problems and to increase stimulation comfort (Szeto 1988). TENS electrodes can now be purchased in a wide variety of sizes and shapes (see Fig. 4.13). These parameters can influence the magnitude and distribution of the current density in the tissues under the electrodes. For a given current, the current density under a small area electrode will be higher and more localised than that under a large area electrode. Small electrodes are therefore well suited to target precisely known points, e.g. motor points. Larger area electrodes tend to distribute the current more evenly and reduce the risk of tissue damage. They are most suitable for stimulating large muscle groups, for example on the lower back. Too large an electrode, however, may cause the current to spread to neighbouring tissues. In some body locations, due, for example, to body contours, it may be difficult to adhere large area electrodes and this could lead to the creation of current density hot spots. This problem can be overcome by the use of several, interconnected, small area electrodes.

The shape of an electrode is another important parameter. It is the shape of the electrode/gel layers rather than the adhesive tape backing which is of interest. The edges of square or rectangular electrodes tend to curl up and the subsequent adhesion of the exposed edge to clothing can then result in the electrodes being peeled off; this problem is minimised with electrodes which are round in shape. The edges of square or rectangular electrodes with angular edges also tend to concentrate the electrical field at these edges, giving rise to current density hot spots. From a manufacturing point of view, depending on the electrode design and the manufacturing process, it is often easier to cut out electrodes in squares or rectangles and this results in less wastage. Rounding off the edges of rectangular electrodes minimises the above problems.

Long rectangular electrodes are often sold in a variety of lengths and widths to be used postoperatively on either side of incisions. Disposable electrodes which are solid gel based can often be cut by the therapist to the size and shape required to stimulate a given target in a given anatomical position. Bow-tie-shaped electrodes are commercially available for applications where square or rectangular electrodes would tend to wrinkle due to the contours of the body.

Electrode attachment

On limbs, electrodes can be held in place using straps or elasticated bands on patients who are sitting or lying down. Belts or harnesses containing TENS electrodes are sometimes used to attach electrodes in their required positions on the torso and may be worn by mobile patients.

Discs or patches of adhesive 'tape' are often

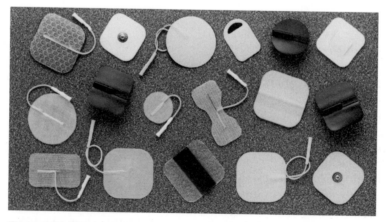

Figure 4.13 Range of electrode designs (Uni-patch Medical Supplies, Wabasha, Minneapolis, USA).

used to hold electrodes in place for relatively long periods of time on many parts of the body. These are suitable for use on mobile patients. Expanded polyester foam tends to give the most secure adhesion. However, as this backing is occlusive, the use of foam can give rise to skin irritation problems. Breathable, cloth-like fabrics allow the transmission of air and moisture and generally cause less skin irritation problems. Cloth-like materials tend to stretch, however (an advantage when it accommodates skin stretching due to movement), and this can lead to the electrode working loose and making poor contact with the skin, possibly resulting in current density hot spots.

Adhesive gels are used in the design of many electrode systems. Such gels help to ensure firm electrical contact between the electrode and the skin, reduce the incidence of current density hot spots and often simplify the design of the electrode. As a large surrounding disc of adhesive tape is not required, the electrode size can be reduced to the 'active' electrode area. The adhesive gel pads can either be replaced (Fig. 4.14), refreshed or simply reused in many semi- or

totally-reusable electrode systems. Conductive 'glues' such as Tac Gel® are sometimes used to attach electrodes to the skin and can be easily removed when necessary.

Electrode design

In the previous sections of this chapter, many aspects of the electrode–gel–skin interface have been overviewed to give the reader a deeper understanding of TENS electrode designs and their proper use. In this section, some of those aspects are brought together and some examples of electrode design for specific applications are given.

In some early forms of electrotherapy (and biosignal monitoring), the electrodes were simply metal buckets or receptacles, filled with water or another electrolyte, into which the subject introduced their foot or hand. Obviously, the range of applications was somewhat limited.

Malleable metal foil electrodes were the next evolutionary step in TENS electrode design. The foil plates were used in conjunction with moistened pads of paper towelling, lint, cotton gauze or sponge. These pads can be moistened by the therapist prior to electrode application with tap water rather than distilled water as the latter is less conductive. Pregelled pads are available and take the form of gel-impregnated sponges or premoistened paper pads. Thicker gel pads are believed to reduce skin irritation problems which result from the by-products of the electrochemical reaction. As this reaction takes place at the electrode–gel interface, the further the skin is distanced from the interface, the better.

Foil plate electrodes are generally held in place with rubber straps or patches, or adhesive tapes/bandages. These electrodes can be readily customised by the therapist and hence are suitable for use in a clinic, especially for applications such as the treatment of low back pain where low cost, large area electrodes may be needed. Due to their inconvenience, such electrodes tend not to be suitable for home-based self-therapy by the patient.

Although electrically more resistive than metal foil electrodes, carbon-loaded rubber elec-

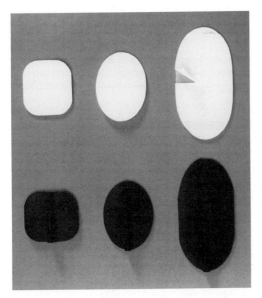

Figure 4.14 Adhesive polymer pads used in conjunction with carbon rubber electrodes (Biomedical Life Systems, California, USA); when they lose their adhesive quality, the pads are simply replaced.

trodes tend to be more convenient to use and are marketed for long term repeated use (Fig. 4.15). They can be made sufficiently thin (while still maintaining their structural integrity and acceptable conductivity) to have high flexibility and thus to be able to conform with body contours. Although generally not cut to shape by the therapist, conductive rubber electrodes can be easily manufactured to just about any size or shape and a wide range of choice exists in the market. The therapist must be aware of possible problems due to uneven current density distribution under the electrodes and to the effects of ageing on the conductivity of the carbon-loaded electrodes.

These electrodes can be used in conjunction with an aqueous electrolyte gel and attached to the patient using elastic straps or custom-cut adhesive patches. Alternatively, conductive, adhesive pads of 'solid' hydrogel may be used to adhere the electrode to the skin and to provide the electrical connection between the electrode and the patient. In this case, the overall area of the electrode is smaller as a surrounding layer of adhesive backing is no longer needed. The entire surface is both conductive and adhesive. In some electrodes, the hydrogel pads can be removed and the conductive rubber electrode cleaned and regelled with a fresh hydrogel pad for further use (Fig. 4.16). In the clinical environment, such a 'semi-reusable' electrode minimises cost and cross-contamination, and is relatively convenient. The hydrogels in some electrodes are dry

and need to be moisture activated prior to use. In certain cases, the electrode can be intermittently reused, on the same patient, by rehydrating the gel pad. Such 'totally-reusable' electrodes are ideal for self-therapy by the home-based patient.

The growing home-based market has led to the great variety of 'low cost' disposable and reusable electrodes which are generally based on solid adhesive gels; such electrodes come in a variety of sizes and shapes (Fig. 4.17) and are easy to apply for home use. 'Snap fastener' electrodes, resembling standard ECG electrodes, are available with sponge discs containing low chloride 'wet' gels. 'Snap fastener' electrodes, with or without a 'current dispersing' conductive

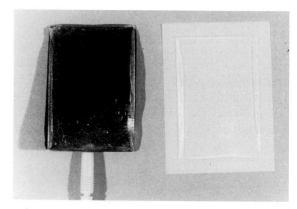

Figure 4.16 Left: Hydrogel pad attached to a carbon rubber electrode. Right: Hydrogel pad between two protective plastic sheets (this is how it is generally supplied).

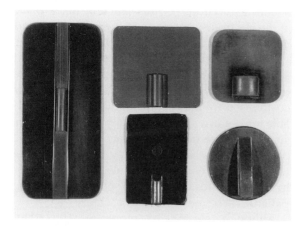

Figure 4.15 Samples of carbon rubber electrodes.

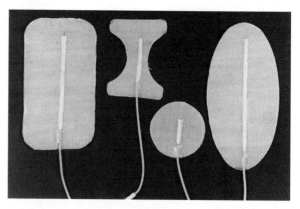

Figure 4.17 Samples of self-adhesive electrodes (Nidd Valley Medical Ltd., North Yorkshire, UK).

sheet, are also available with relatively larger hydrogel pads.

Electrodes are also made using conductive cloth-like materials; thin metallic foils; aluminised carbon-filled mylar; or wire strands. Electrical connection is generally made to these electrodes via alligator clips, snap fasteners or pin connectors (Fig. 4.18). Some have integrated lead wires with 'pig tail' connectors and thus the electrodes are not connected directly to the TENS unit's leads (Fig. 4.17). An advantage of this

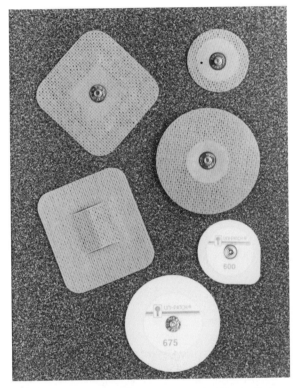

Figure 4.18 Top: Four pregelled electrodes constructed with breathable cloth backing. Bottom: Two pregelled electrodes constructed of moisture-resistant foam backing. (From Uni-patch Medical Supplies, PO Box 271, 1313 West Grant Boulevard, Wabasha, MN 55981, USA.)

design is that the electrodes can be connected/disconnected to the unit without disturbing the electrode–skin interface.

Many of these hydrogel-based electrodes can be trimmed to the desired size or shape by simply cutting with a pair of scissors.

Postoperative TENS electrodes must be sterile and convenient to apply. A pregelled, disposable electrode is therefore best suited for this purpose. Such electrodes tend to be long foil/hydrogel electrodes and are supplied in sterile packages. Postoperative electrodes generally have relatively long integrated leads to distance the TENS unit's leads from the sterile electrodes.

SUMMARY OF KEY POINTS

1. The science pertaining to TENS electrodes is far from simple and a large number of inter-related factors must be understood if a TENS device is to be operated successfully without trauma to the patient.

2. Constant current devices with voltage limitations are highly recommended from a safety point of view.

3. The electrical properties of the outer layers of the skin form the major component of the overall lead–electrode–patient system.

4. The distribution of current density under an electrode will influence the efficacy of treatment and is an important factor in skin irritation.

5. There are many different commercially available electrode designs. The design best suited for a given application will depend on the anatomical location to be treated, the length of the treatment, whether the treatment is to be carried out in a clinic or in the patient's own home, the sensitivity of the patient to the various sources of skin irritation, financial constraints, etc.

REFERENCES

Campbell J A 1982 A critical appraisal of the electrical output characteristics of TENS transcutaneous nerve stimulators. Clinical Physiological Measurement 3: 141–150
Carim H M 1988 Bioelectrodes. In: Webster J G (ed)

Encyclopedia of medical devices and instrumentation. Wiley, New York
Caruso P M, Pearce J A, DeWitt D P 1979 Temperature and current density distributions at electrosurgical

dispersive electrode sites. Proceedings of the 7th New England Bioengineering Conference, pp. 373–376

Cook T M 1987 Instrumentation. In: Nelson R M, Currier D P (eds) Clinical electrotherapy. Appleton and Lange, Connecticutt

Cromwell L, Arditti M, Weibell F J, Pfeiffer E A, Steele B, Labok J 1976 Medical instrumentation for health care. Prentice Hall, New Jersey

Low J, Reed A 1994 Electrotherapy explained: principles and practice. Butterworth-Heinemann, Oxford

McAdams E T, Jossinet J 1991 The importance of electrode–skin impedance in high resolution electrocardiography. Automedica 13: 187–208

McAdams E T, Henry P, Anderson J 1992 Optimal electrolytic chloriding of silver ink electrodes for use in electrical impedance tomography. Clinical Physics and

Physiological Measurement 13: A19–23

McAdams E T, Lackermeier A, McLaughlin J A, Macken D 1995 The linear and non-linear electrical properties of the electrode–electrolyte interface. Biosensors and Bioelectronics 10: 67–74

Mannheimer J S, Lampe G N 1984 Clinical transcutaneous electrical nerve stimulation. F A Davis, Philadelphia

Reilly J P 1992 Electrical stimulation and electropathology. Cambridge University Press, Cambridge

Szeto A Y J 1988 Pain relief using transcutaneous electrical nerve stimulation (TENS). In: Webster J G (ed) Encyclopedia of medical devices and instrumentation. Wiley, New York

Yamamoto Y, Yamamoto T 1978 Dispersion and correlation of the parameters for skin impedance. Medical and Biological Engineering and Computing 16: 592–594

Introduction   63

Neurophysiological studies   64
Animal studies   64
Human studies   68
   Summary   70

Experimental pain studies   70
   Classes of experimental pain methods   71
Thermal pain   71
Mechanical pain   75
Ischaemic pain   76
Delayed onset muscle soreness (DOMS)   76
Cold-induced pain   77
Electrical pain   78
   Experimental pain model criteria   79

Summary of key points   79

5

Review of experimental studies on TENS

INTRODUCTION

This chapter will focus on the experimental or laboratory-based studies that have been completed on TENS. Whereas some may consider laboratory studies to be insignificant with regard to the clinical application of TENS, it should be remembered that they have the potential to provide useful data upon which to base TENS treatment regimes. Furthermore, if such studies are performed in a controlled and systematic manner they can serve as an essential prerequisite to clinical trials. In addition, these non-clinical studies can help to determine the precise mechanism of action of TENS. A number of criteria can be used to judge the quality of a laboratory study:

1. Is there a stable laboratory environment, i.e. are noise, temperature, etc. controlled?

2. Are sufficient details provided on the methodology employed? Can the study be easily replicated?

3. Was a control and/or placebo group included for comparison with the treatment group?

4. Was the output of the treatment under investigation tested? Quite often the output of a machine does not correspond with the readings obtained from an appropriate measuring apparatus. It is always important to calibrate an apparatus prior to conducting an experiment so that precise details of treatment parameters can be given (see Ch. 3 for details on how to calibrate the output of a TENS unit).

With the above criteria in mind, the most

pertinent experimental work completed on TENS to date will be discussed under two headings – neurophysiological studies and experimental pain studies.

NEUROPHYSIOLOGICAL STUDIES

Neurophysiological studies involve recording neural activity either peripherally from an individual nerve fibre or an entire nerve, centrally from a plexus of nerves (e.g. Erbs point evoked potential) or from the scalp (e.g. somatosensory evoked potential). The information obtained from such studies can provide an insight into whether a modality affects nerve conduction and if so, at what stage of the neural pathway the effect occurs. A summary of the most relevant in vitro and in vivo experimental studies on the neurophysiological effects of electrical stimulation completed to date is presented in Table 5.1. This table highlights the range of stimulation parameters used and the variability of results obtained.

In the following neurophysiological studies, reference will be made to different characteristics of the compound action potential (CAP) which are used as objective data for statistical analyses. For the purposes of clarification for the reader, these characteristics are illustrated on a schematic diagram of a CAP in Figure 5.1. The animal

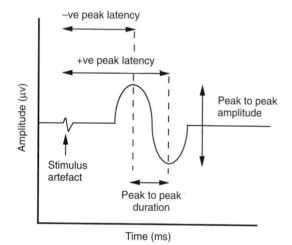

Figure 5.1 Schematic diagram of a compound action potential.

and human neurophysiological studies will now be discussed separately.

Animal studies

Neurophysiological studies in animals permit recording from dissected nerves, a technique which would not be ethically permissible in humans. The majority of animal work completed to date has involved in vivo and in vitro studies on cats and rats; these studies have, for the most part, focused on changes in peripheral neural activity post electrical stimulation. Ignelzi & Nyquist (1976) investigated the effect of electrical currents of variable frequency, intensity and duration on isolated cat superficial radial and sural nerves (the central attachments of the nerves were severed, isolating them from the central nervous system). In this study, the electrical current was delivered via a cuff stimulator positioned around the isolated nerve. The results showed that in seven out of 10 experiments, there was either a decrease in amplitude or an increase in latency in the Aα, Aβ and A∂ CAP waves (an increase in latency corresponds to a decrease in conduction velocity).

The observed changes were found to be reversible and occurred to a greater extent in the A∂ component of the CAP. These changes in latency and amplitude are indicative of some interruption of activity in these fibre types. Based upon these results, the authors suggest that the application of electrical currents may produce a block of conduction in peripheral nerve fibres. It is assumed that the authors are referring to a decrease in conduction velocity when they refer to a 'block of conduction' and not a complete block which indicates absence of the CAP. The term 'peripheral block' is used in several places throughout this chapter and the former interpretation will be ascribed to it.

This work was extended in 1979 (Ignelzi & Nyquist 1979a) to investigate the excitability changes in single nerve fibres of the cat superficial radial nerve following repetitive electrical stimulation. In this study, a relatively high frequency (180–200/sec) was used and current increased to threshold intensity. The results of

Table 5.1 Neurophysiological studies on TENS

Reference	Species	n	Stimulation	Duration	Placebo	Record	Effect
Campbell & Taub 1973	Human	6	50 V, 100 Hz, 0.5 ms (i) continuous (ii) periodic	?	No	CAP median nerve	Cont stim-dec in amp & inc in lat Aα wave, dec in Aδ wave – ? peripheral blockade
Torebjörk & Hallin 1974	Human	6	Square wave 50–100 μs, 0.5–100 Hz	?	No	Microelectrodes in radial nerve	Increase in latency of both A and C unit responses
Ignelzi & Nyquist 1976	Cat	10	Variable frequency, intensity and duration	1s–30'	No	CAP from isolated sural and superficial radial nerves	Reversible changes in Aα, Aβ and Aδ waves; 7/10 showed dec amp or inc latency of these waves; Aδ showed gtr changes – ? fibre block
Worth & Ochs 1976	Cat	11	~350 pps	1–3 hours	Control	Fast axoplasmic transport in the sciatic nerve	15% dec (sig) in rate of fast axoplasmic transport following electrical stimulation
Ignelzi & Nyquist 1979a	Cat	85 fibres	Square wave 180–200/sec, 0.2 ms threshold intensity	5–20'	Control n = 364	CAP from single superficial radial nerve fibres	88% underwent excitability changes ? peripheral blocking of fibres
Ignelzi & Nyquist 1979b	Cat	13	(i) 200 pps, < 1.3 mA (ii) 280/350 pps 8–10X CAP threshold 0.2 ms	5/6 hours	Control	CAP and fast axoplasmic transport in the sciatic nerve	Dec in CAP, no effect on fast axoplasmic transport
Janko & Trontelj 1980	Human	8	Rectangular and triangular pulses 0.1–3 ms, variable Hz	?	No	Microneurography median, ulnar and radial nerves	Inc stimulus freq-inc jitter and intermittent blocking of spike components
Salar et al 1980	Human	6	Square wave, 60 Hz 200 μs, 40–80 m	15'	No	Late + ive SEP median nerve	Sig dec in amp of P50–60 component during TENS
Ignelzi et al 1981	Cat	80 fibres	Square wave, 0.2 ms 1–14 V, 6–200 Hz	5–30'	No	Discharge of SC cells and DC fibres (sciatic nerve)	46% – suppressive effect 36% – no influence 5% – transient facilitatory change
Francini et al 1981	Human	65	Rectangular, 50 Hz, 1 ms constant tingling	24–40'	No	H & Achilles tendon reflexes Cutaneous pain threshold	Relationship between sensory thresholds and reflex responses. Changes more marked in pain patients than healthy subjects
Francini et al 1982	Human	19	Square wave, 50 Hz, 1 ms tingling sensation	25'	No	SEP median nerve	Changes in amp of late SEP components
Ashton et al 1984a	Human	32	100 Hz, 200 μs strong, comfortable	~45'	Yes	Late SEPs	Sig inc N1 lat, sig dec N1P2 amp Sig dec SEP total excursion
Chung et al 1984a	Monkey	46	2 Hz, Int = 200–300x threshold of largest A fibres	15'	No	STT cell activity	Inhibition of STT cells
Chung et al 1984b	Monkey	19	0.5–20 Hz varying intensities	5'	No	STT cell activity	Frequency and intensity specific inhibition of STT cells

Table 5.1 (contd)

Reference	Species	n	Stimulation	Duration	Placebo	Record	Effect
Katims & Ng 1985	Rat	12	Sinusoid wave 5/2000 Hz, 0.25 mA PPA	?	Control	Autoradiographs, metabolic activity in the brain	Substantial localised inc in CNS metabolic activity in TENS groups
Sjölund 1985	Rat	82	Monophasic square 10–160 Hz, 150 ms (i) 2x threshold (ii) 10x threshold	30'	No	C-fibre evoked flexion reflex	Depression of reflex 10x threshold (40–160 Hz all sig) was more effective than 2x threshold (80–100 Hz more effective)
Golding et al 1986	Human	26	100 Hz, 200 µs strong, comfortable	30'	Yes	SEP	Sig dec amp early and late SEP
Walmsley et al 1986	Human	12	100 Hz, 100 µs mild, tingling	30'	No	Sensory cond vel and skin temp median nerve	Sig dec in cond vel / Sig dec in skin temp
Chan & Tsang 1987	Human	11	Square wave, 100 Hz 1 ms, subj tingling	30'	Yes	EMG of flexion reflex in BF, TA and HF	Depression of flexion reflex – gradual onset and offset
Cox et al 1993	Human	31	Square wave 2/85 Hz, 100/250 µs 24.4/26.7 mA	20'	Yes	Motor cond vel and skin temp ulnar nerve	No sig effect on cond vel or skin temp
Hui-Chan & Levin 1993	Human	10	Square wave, 99 Hz, 0.125 ms, 2x sensory threshold	45'	Yes	H and stretch reflexes Soleus	Inc in H and stretch reflexes in TENS groups applied seg and heteroseg / Placebo – no effect
Levin & Hui-Chan 1993	Human	17	Conv T-3x threshold Acu T (i) 0.1 Hz (ii) 100 Hz–4 Hz trains	?	No	CAP median nerve	Mainly Aαβ fibres activated by TENS
Walsh et al 1995a	Human	40	Asymm biphasic 4/110 Hz, 50/200 µs strong, comfortable	15'	Control	CAP and skin temp superficial radial nerve	Sig inc NPL 110 Hz, 200 µs group
Walsh et al 1995b	Human	24	Asymm biphasic 110 Hz/200 µs, 4 Hz/50 µs strong, comfortable	15'	Control	CAP and skin temp superficial radial nerve	Sig inc NPL 110 Hz, 200 µs group Inc in NPL lasted up to 30' post TENS

Abbreviations:
Amp = amplitude; **BF** = biceps femoris; **CAP** = compound action potential; **CNS** = central nervous system; **DC** = dorsal column; **Dec** = decrease; **Freq** = frequency; **HF** = hip flexors; **Inc** = increase; **Lat** = latency; **TA** = tibialis anterior; **SC** = spinal cord; **SEP** = somatosensory evoked potential.

this study confirmed their previous observations: 88% of the 85 preparations showed an excitability change upon termination of repetitive electrical stimulation. The predominant change observed in 82% of the preparations was a decrease in excitability manifested as a transient decrease in conduction velocity and/or an increase in electrical threshold for discharge. Again, the authors proposed an 'unselective' or generalised blocking of large fibre afferent inflow by high frequency repetitive stimulation; similar excitability changes appeared to occur in fibres of both large and small diameter. This proposal is not consistent with Melzack & Wall's gate control theory (i.e. small diameter fibre activity is reduced by large diameter fibre activity; Melzack & Wall 1965), as such suppression of large fibre activity would result in decreased ability to inhibit nociceptive input at a spinal segmental level.

The same researchers subsequently studied the effect of repetitive electrical stimulation of the sciatic nerve on the discharge of spinal cord cells and dorsal column fibres on 80 intact preparations of the anaesthetised cat (Ignelzi et al 1981). This study showed that 46% of spinal cord units showed inhibited or depressed discharge following 5–30 minutes of repetitive electrical stimulation. Transient facilitated discharge was observed in 5% of units, while 36% showed no influence. This study indicated that the peripheral suppression following repetitive electrical stimulation observed in previous experiments (described above) was reflected in altered discharge activity at the spinal cord. Ignelzi's group has logically progressed their work from peripheral nerve recording to central recording from dorsal horn fibres; at both levels, a suppression of neural activity was observed.

Chung et al (1984a) reported an inhibition of spinothalamic tract (STT) cell activity in the monkey after 15 minutes of 2 Hz high intensity stimulation of a peripheral nerve. In a similar experiment on STT cell activity, this group investigated the effect of different intensities and frequencies of the conditioning stimulus applied to a peripheral nerve (5 minutes, 0.5–20 Hz) upon inhibition of these cells (Chung et al 1984b). It was reported that using intensities sufficient to

stimulate the A∂ fibre group was more effective in producing inhibition of the STT cells compared to intensities required to stimulate the A$\alpha\beta$ or C fibre groups. In addition, it was noted that the higher the frequency used at a fixed intensity, the greater the inhibition of STT cells. This study has therefore highlighted the varying effects of both intensity and frequency of peripheral stimulation upon STT cells.

The effect of electrical stimulation on other aspects of neural function has also been investigated in animals. The application of sinusoidal TENS to the ears of rats has been shown to alter CNS metabolic activity (Katims & Ng 1985). Two stimulation frequencies were used in this study (5 Hz and 2000 Hz), both of which caused localised increases in CNS metabolic activity compared to controls. Interestingly, the lower frequency caused a comparatively greater increase in metabolic activity in the region of the nuclei ambiguii and trigeminal nuclei (analysed by autoradiographs), whereas the 2000 Hz group appeared to selectively increase activity in the region of the nucleus solitarius and vestibular nuclei. This study suggests that a sinusoidal TENS current can selectively excite different neuronal populations depending upon the frequency selected.

The effect of repetitive stimulation of cat sciatic nerve on fast axoplasmic transport has been investigated by Ignelzi & Nyquist (1979b). This mechanism is responsible for the peripheral transport of proteins and other vital neural constituents which are synthesised in the neuronal soma. Even when the CAP was almost abolished following repetitive electrical stimulation, there was no effect on the rate of fast axoplasmic transport. Stimulation parameters used in this study were in the range commonly used in clinical practice (200 p/sec, 0.2 ms). This might suggest that the observed effects are not due to a decrease in transport of essential substrates within the nerve.

In contrast, a similar study by Worth & Ochs (1976) reported a 15% decrease in the rate of axoplasmic transport in cat sciatic nerves following electrical stimulation. Repetitive electrical stimulation ~350 pps applied for 1–3 hours, produced a significant (p < 0.01) reduction in transport rate, compared with control values. The current intensities used in this study were not given which makes comparison of the two studies difficult. In addition, this work was carried out in vitro, which meant that there was an irreplaceable depletion of energy substrates. The blood supply was intact in Ignelzi & Nyquist's study and therefore there was a constant supply of ATP, which is necessary for the axoplasmic transport mechanism.

In contrast to the above, the work of Sjölund (1985) was directed at determining the optimal parameters of a current applied to a cutaneous nerve to maximally suppress the C-fibre-evoked flexion reflex elicited in a nearby spinal segment. Monophasic square wave pulses were applied to the plantar and sural nerves of the rat for a 30-minute period. The common peroneal and sciatic nerves were exposed for flexion reflex/nerve volley recordings. In this study, frequency and intensity-specific effects were noted. At 10 times threshold intensity (i.e the intensity that just gave a barely visible nerve volley in the sciatic nerve) a range of frequencies (40–160 Hz) produced significant depression of the reflex. However, when only twice threshold intensity was applied, only those frequencies between 80 and 100 Hz caused a marked depression. The authors suggest a clinical application of these results in the selection of stimulation parameters, e.g. combining high intensities with frequencies above 100 Hz and lower intensities with frequencies in the 80–100 Hz range.

Although some interesting results have been obtained from the animal neurophysiological studies discussed in this section, the difficulties in extrapolating effective stimulation parameters to the human model remains a problem. Thus, it appears that human neurophysiological studies represent better models for the investigation of electrical stimulation.

Human studies

The human studies in Table 5.1 have concentrated on two types of neurophysiological recordings from the neural axis:

- the peripheral nerve CAP
- centrally evoked potentials.

Initial studies tended to focus on whether electrical stimulation produced an effect or not, whereas more recent studies have introduced the element of parameter manipulation into the experimental procedure. One of the earliest studies of note was performed by Campbell & Taub (1973), who investigated the effect of periodic and continuous stimulation of the median nerve. Digital electrodes were used to deliver the electrical stimulation (50 V, 100 Hz, 0.5 ms) and the CAP was recorded at wrist. After a period of adaptation (~20 minutes), the median nerve CAP showed a decrease in amplitude and increase in latency of the Aα wave and a decrease in A∂ wave; this was observed only when stimulation was continuous. The authors consequently suggested that a conduction block occurred following such percutaneous stimulation. This result also questions the physiological basis of Melzack & Wall's gate control theory as it would appear that the large diameter fibres are being suppressed rather than stimulated when the high frequency electrical current is applied.

Using the same nerve, Walmsley et al (1986) similarly reported that 30 minutes of TENS (100 Hz, 100 μs) produced a significant decrease in sensory conduction velocity, although no control group was used in this study to compare changes over time in the resting subject. More recently and in contrast, Cox et al (1993) reported no significant change in human ulnar motor nerve conduction velocity following the application of either acupuncture-like (2 Hz, 250 μs) or conventional (85 Hz, 100 μs) TENS.

Walsh et al (1995a) have demonstrated a significant increase in conduction latency in the superficial radial nerve following the application of TENS for a 15-minute period (three consecutive 5-minute periods); this study produced a novel finding in that it was also found that the observed neurophysiological effect was dependent upon the combinations of pulse frequency and pulse duration parameters used. The stimulation parameters employed were four combinations from the upper and lower extremes of range of pulse frequency (4 Hz and 110 Hz) and pulse duration (50 μs and 200 μs) commonly used in clinical practice. The 110 Hz, 200 μs TENS group showed a statistically significant increase in latency compared to the control group. A more recent extension of this study (Walsh et al 1995b) has additionally demonstrated that the increase in latency in this TENS group was evident for up to 30 minutes after the TENS unit was switched off.

Somatosensory evoked potentials (SEPs) are potentials elicited by stimulation of peripheral nerves and recorded by electrodes placed on the scalp. SEPs are consequently smaller in amplitude and longer in latency than the compound action potentials recorded from a peripheral nerve. The amplitude of the late components of the SEP has been proposed as an objective neurophysiological correlate of pain and hypoalgesia (Ashton et al 1984a). Golding et al (1986) further suggest that early components of SEPs are likely to represent cortical processing from Aα fibres, and the late SEPs cortical processing from Aβ and A∂ afferents. A study conducted by this group showed that following 30 minutes of TENS (100 Hz, 200 μs) application over the median nerve at the wrist (the side of TENS application was randomised), a significant decrease in amplitude of both early and late components was observed in the SEP (recorded from both mastoids, FZ', CZ, C3', ˙C4'). However, the authors reported that in a separate experiment, application of TENS showed no attenuation of evoked potentials recorded at the elbow. They therefore conclude that the site of action of TENS may be spinal, subcortical, cortical or a combination of levels and dismiss the importance of a peripheral effect.

Ashton et al (1984a) used a similar experimental procedure to compare the application of TENS over the median nerve (45 minutes) to the effect of aspirin on late SEPs (recorded from CZ and linked mastoids). In their analysis using difference scores, it was found that the N_1P_2 amplitude significantly decreased and the N_1 latency significantly increased in the TENS group, compared to either the placebo or aspirin groups; this effect was observed immediately post TENS. In ad-

dition, the SEP total excurs[...] creased with TENS at the [...] stimulation; there was als[...] the 45-minute point.

Evoked potential techniques have also [...] used by Salar et al (1980), who reported a significant decrease in amplitude of the late positive component of the SEP (recorded from both parietal lobes) following application of TENS (60 Hz, 200 μs) for 15 minutes over the median nerve at the wrist. When intravenous naloxone (an opiate antagonist) was administered, there was a reversal of the hypoalgesia induced by TENS in four out of the six subjects studied. However, after the administration of intravenous saline, there was no change in the SEP. Furthermore, in these four subjects there was a significant increase in amplitude of the late positive component in the SEP. This reversal of hypoalgesia by naloxone would suggest that the opiate system plays some part in the observed TENS-mediated neurophysiological effects. An increase in the number of subjects used in this study would have been useful to provide more power in the statistical analysis.

Francini et al (1982) studied the relevance of the site of application of TENS on SEPs (recorded from the right scalp 3 cm behind C3–C4). TENS (50 Hz, 1 ms) was applied over the median nerve on both sides. They found that TENS produced changes in the amplitude of the late SEP components, independent of whether it was applied contralateral or ipsilateral to the evoking stimuli. In contrast, Golding et al (1986) found that the changes observed in their study (already discussed) were largely confined to SEPs generated from the hand treated with TENS (i.e. ipsilateral side).

The effect of TENS on human flexion reflexes in the lower limb has also been studied (Chan & Tsang 1987). This group applied TENS (100 Hz, 1 ms) paravertebrally at the level of L4–S1 for 30 minutes. Electromyography (EMG) recordings were taken from the tibialis anterior, biceps femoris and hip flexor muscles. It was observed that TENS produced a progressive depression of the flexion reflex that took ~10–30 minutes to reach a peak and that outlasted the stimulation for riable periods (up to 50 minutes). This pattern was observed in the majority of the 11 subjects examined and it was noted that the inhibitory effect was more prominent on the proximal than distal lower limb muscles.

Similarly, Francini et al (1981) studied the changes induced by TENS on the H-reflex and the Achilles tendon reflex in both healthy and chronic myofascial pain subjects. TENS (1 ms, 50 Hz) was applied over the posterior surface of the leg (cathode) and the anterior surface of the leg (anode) for periods of up to 40 minutes. Results showed an interesting relationship between the pain threshold of the subject and the changes induced in the reflexes; when the pain threshold before TENS application was low, it was found that TENS induced an inhibitory effect on both the afferent and efferent components of the reflex; when the threshold was high the effect was mainly facilitatory. Furthermore, these changes were more marked in the chronic myofascial pain subjects than in healthy subjects.

In a similar study on reflexes, Hui-Chan & Levin (1993) reported an increase in both the soleus H-reflex and stretch reflex latencies following TENS application (both segmentally and heterosegmentally) in spastic hemiparetic subjects. The authors postulated that such effects may be mediated by $A\alpha\beta$ fibres as a previous study by the same authors had concluded that both conventional and acupuncture-like TENS stimulate mainly these fibre types (Levin & Hui-Chan 1993).

Finally, microneurographic techniques have also been employed to investigate the neurophysiological effects of electrical stimulation. This invasive technique involves selective recording of neural activity from thin electrodes inserted into the nerves. Janko & Trontelj (1980) applied triangular and rectangular shaped electrical pulses via digital ring electrodes and recorded activity in the ulnar, median and radial nerves above the wrist. They noted that increases in stimulus frequency usually resulted in increased jitter (i.e. latency variation of consecutive responses) as well as intermittent blocking of some spike components. The increased jitter erroneously resulted in decreased amplitude and appearance of false spikes in the averaged recording. The authors maintained that this was due to a technical artefact and not a true reflection of the activity in the nerves. They therefore dismissed the role of peripheral mechanisms in the neurophysiological effects of TENS. This study therefore reported no differences between the two waveforms in terms of the activity elicited in the peripheral nerves by each.

Torebjörk & Hallin (1974) used microelectrodes inserted into the radial nerve to record the A and C fibre response to repeated intradermal electrical stimulation (50–100 µs, 0.5–100 pulses/s). This experiment found a progressive, frequency-dependent increase in latency of both A and especially C components to repetitive electrical stimulation; as a consequence, the authors concluded that excitation failure in peripheral thin nerve fibres may be responsible for the decrease in pain perception observed during repetitive intradermal stimulation at high frequencies.

Summary

In summary, the majority of the human neurophysiological studies discussed in this section have reported significant changes in neurophysiological function at both a peripheral and cortical level as a result of the peripheral application of electrical stimulation. It is probably not surprising that application of an electrical current from a stimulator could alter electrical activity (that is, action potentials) in a nerve. What is surprising is that combinations of parameters can produce completely different effects (Walsh et al 1995a) and this observation calls for further microneurographic investigations to determine which fibres are affected.

EXPERIMENTAL PAIN STUDIES

When any new modality comes onto the market claiming to produce pain relief, it is invariably met with a degree of scepticism. The analgesic efficacy of the modality can be subsequently determined by its effectiveness on both experimental and clinical models of pain. As the primary effect of TENS is analgesia, it therefore follows that experimental pain will be employed to examine the analgesic efficacy of TENS using a variety of models. In this section, a detailed account is provided of a selection of studies which have reported the effects of TENS on experimental pain. Experimental pain studies, used to determine the analgesic potential of various agents, have developed considerably over the past 50 years. Gracely (1991) outlines the main advantages of experimental methods for evaluating analgesic efficacy as follows:

- They are less expensive and statistically more powerful than clinical trials. Problems involved in conducting a clinical trial include staff and patient recruitment, obtaining ethical approval, coping with non-compliance and drop-out, all of which can prove to be an enormous burden.
- Fast efficient evaluations can be obtained under controlled conditions.

Although experimental models may oversimplify the complex processes of clinical pain, they do allow some quantitative control which is not present in clinical pain (Woolf 1979); the duration and intensity of experimental pain are controlled and subjects are aware of its finite nature, whereas the temporal and intensity boundaries of clinical pain cannot be manipulated. For these various reasons, experimental studies can be viewed as a useful prerequisite to clinical studies provided an appropriate model of pain is used.

The use of animals in experimental studies permits the manipulation of physiological variables which would be ethically impossible in humans, thus important information can be obtained from experimental pain studies in animals which investigate the analgesic effects of a given agent. This information is, however, limited by the difficulties in extrapolating an effective dosage for the human species. In addition, only indirect signs of pain (e.g. withdrawal or autonomic reactions) may be observed in animal studies, whereas in human studies a verbal report is also obtainable (Procacci et al 1979). Therefore, in this review of experimental pain, only human models are considered whereas in the neurophysiology review both animal and human models have been included.

Classes of experimental pain methods

Over the years, a variety of experimental pain models have been developed to investigate the efficacy of analgesic drugs and therapeutic modalities. However, there are essentially three main classes of laboratory pain-induction method (see Wolff 1977):

1. Cutaneous. As the term implies, this method involves the application of a noxious stimulus to the skin. A variety of stimuli have been used to produce cutaneous experimental pain; these stimuli may be thermal, electrical, chemical or mechanical in origin.
2. Deep somatic. This method relates to the stimulation of deep somatic structures, e.g. bone, muscle and periosteum.
3. Visceral. This method involves the stimulation of visceral structures such as the stomach and bladder.

Of the three classes of experimental pain listed above, the first two have routinely been used in the experimental study of the analgesic effects of TENS with thermal, mechanical, ischaemic, cold-induced and electrical pain and delayed onset muscle soreness used as typical models. In the following subsections, each of these types of experimental pain model will be discussed in terms of the results obtained with TENS and the effectiveness of the model. Table 5.2 provides a summary of the main human experimental pain studies that have been completed to date in this area. As can be seen from this table, in addition to simply assessing hypoalgesic efficacy, a number of these studies have also compared the effects of different stimulation frequencies, intensities and types of output on experimental pain. It is encouraging to note that the relevance of stimulation parameters to hypoalgesic effects are being tested by some workers, not least because this was one of the areas of ambiguity highlighted by the survey of chartered physiotherapists described in Chapter 1.

Thermal pain

Of the studies reviewed, thermal pain applied in a variety of ways was the most commonly used

Table 5.2 Experimental pain studies and TENS

Reference	Model of pain	n	Stimulation	Duration	Groups	Results
Campbell & Taub, 1973	Needle stimuli	11	Square wave, 100 Hz, 1 ms, 10–12 V or 22 V	?	2	10–12 V inc in touch threshold only / 22 V sig inc touch and pain thresholds
Woolf 1979	Thermal mechanical & ischaemic	80	Square wave 100 Hz, 0.25 ms variable intensity (2–20 V)	30'+	Placebo Control 3 TENS	Thermal P – high intensity TENS sig inc thermal pain threshold and tolerance / Mechanical P – no effect / Ischaemic P – TENS sig inc in tolerance time and dec in VAS readings
Pertovaara 1980	Thermal	6	Biphasic impulses 100 Hz, 35 mA/45 mA	?	Control TENS	Sig inc in thermal pain threshold when thermal stimuli placed distal to TENS at 45 mA
Sagers & Byrd 1983	Radiant heat CFPT	60	Continuous hyperstimulation	2'	Control TENS	Sig inc in radiant heat CFPT following TENS
Ashton et al 1984b	Cold-induced	46	8 Hz (5.45 mA) 100 Hz (9.1 mA), 200 µs strong but comfortable	50'	Placebo Acupuncture 2 TENS	Ice pain threshold – 8 Hz (no sig) and acupuncture (sig) produced a marked overall increase / Ice pain tolerance – sig inc with 8 Hz and acupuncture
Roche et al 1984	Ischaemic	48	Square wave Cont – 100 Hz, 1 ms Train – 5 Hz, 100 ms 3.7–14.2 V High/non-noxious int or perceptible pricking	10' tolerance reported	Control 3 TENS	Pain endurance – only effectively increased with high int cont TENS / Pain tolerance – sig inc with high int cont and low int train TENS / Pain threshold – sig inc with low int train TENS VAS & PPI – no sig differences with TENS
Eriksson et al 1985	Thermal	8	80 Hz, 2–3 × threshold 2 Hz, 3–5 × threshold	15'	2 TENS	Dec thermal sensitivity in 6/8 subjects / Similar results with both modes / Contralateral and ipsilateral TENS produced the same results
Oliveri et al 1986	Electrical	45	Auricular TENS monophasic, 1 Hz highest tolerated int	90 s per point × 4 points	Control 2 TENS app and inapp auricular points	Sig inc in pain threshold in app auricular TENS only
Jette 1987	Exercise-induced	28	85 Hz & 2 Hz High int (tolerance) Low int (perceptible)	20'	4 TENS	TENS dec (no sig) muscle soreness / Greatest effect observed during treatment
Denegar & Huff 1988	DOMS	24	(i) 80 pps, ~90 µs, monophasic (ii) 2 pps, 200 µs, biphasic	30'	4 TENS	Sig dec in perceived pain across time / No overall differences between (i) and (ii) types of stimulation
Noling et al 1988	Electrical	45	Auricular TENS monophasic, 1 Hz highest tolerated int	90 s per point × 4 points	Control 2 TENS app and inapp auricular points	Sig inc in pain threshold in app auricular TENS only
Denegar et al 1989	DOMS	8	2 Hz, 300 µs max tolerance	30'	TENS	Sig dec in pain perception

Table 5.2 (contd)

REVIEW OF EXPERIMENTAL STUDIES ON TENS 73

Reference	Model of pain	n	Stimulation	Duration	Groups	Results
Johnson et al 1989	Cold-induced	83	10, 20, 40, 80 and 160 Hz, 200 μs, varied int 4.62–5.71 mA strong but comfortable	50'	Placebo Control 7 TENS	Ice pain threshold – sig inc combined TENS vs control/plac, greatest inc observed in freq 20–80 Hz Ice pain tolerance – no sig differences
Johnson et al 1991a	Cold-induced	84	80 Hz, 200 μs burst, modulation, random and cont outputs 4.76–18.7 mA strong but comfortable	50'	Control 5 TENS	Ice pain threshold – sig inc combined TENS vs control cont output showed greatest inc Ice pain tolerance – all outputs inc (no sig), greatest inc in cont output
Johnson et al 1991b	Electrical	24	2.3 Hz trains, 100 Hz within trains strong, comfortable	15'	Auricular TENS Control 3 TENS	Electrical pain threshold – no sig difference between combined TENS and control Autonomic variables – no sig differences
Marchand et al 1991	Thermal	7	100 Hz, 125 μs, clear but non painful paraesthesia	25'	Placebo TENS	Heat pain threshold – sig inc during and post TENS. TENS sig dec ratings of painful and near painful heat stimuli
Johnson et al 1992	Cold-induced	60	5 TENS modes described	30'	4 TENS Placebo	All modes small, insig effect on pain intensity Variable effect on pain threshold depending on mode and intensity
Taylor et al 1993	Electrical	72	Sine-wave constant AC monophasic 5/100/2000 Hz Int = 0.05 mA below current perception threshold	30'	Auricular TENS 3 TENS Placebo	Sig inc trig nerve sensation threshold post active TENS with 5 and 100 Hz producing greatest hypoaesthesia
Walsh et al 1995a	Mechanical	48	Asymm biphasic 4/110 Hz, 50/200 μs strong, comfortable	15'	4 TENS Placebo Control	Sig and greatest inc in MPT in 110 Hz, 200 μs TENS group
Walsh et al 1995c	Ischaemic	32	Asymm biphasic 4/110 Hz, 287 μs strong, comfortable	22'	2 TENS Placebo Control	Sig dec in mean VAS – 4 Hz TENS Sig dec VAS diff scores – 4 Hz TENS No sig diff in MPQ

Abbreviations:
App = appropriate; CFPT = C fibre pain threshold; Cont = continuous; Dec = decrease; Diff = difference; Inapp = Inappropriate; Inc = increase; Int = intensity; MPQ = McGill Pain Questionnaire; MPT = mechanical pain threshold; P = pain; Plac = placebo; Sig = significant; VAS = visual analogue scale.

type of experimental pain (Eriksson et al 1985, Marchand et al 1991, Pertovaara 1980, Sagers & Byrd 1983, Woolf 1979). Thermal pain was one of the three types of experimental pain used by Woolf (1979) to investigate electrical stimulation hypoalgesia. In this study, thermal pain was applied by water which was circulated at a controlled temperature through a circular capsule held in contact with the forearm. This capsule was used to test pain threshold and tolerance (i.e. the time it took for the subject to report the thermal sensation reaching a painful level, and subsequently, when they could no longer tolerate it). The TENS electrodes were positioned for maximal stimulation of the median nerve (the authors did not indicate exact positioning of electrodes). TENS (100 Hz, 0.25 ms) was applied for 30 minutes before and during the testing procedure, and stimulation intensities ranged from 'low' to 'very high' (2–20 V). The high intensity TENS group (20 V) showed significant elevations of both pain threshold (p < 0.01) and pain tolerance (p < 0.05); these increases were not observed in the placebo nor in the two lower intensity TENS groups (2 V or 10 V). By showing the best (and in fact the only) significant effect in the high intensity TENS group, this study highlighted the relevance of stimulation intensity in TENS-mediated hypoalgesia.

Experimental pain studies using thermal pain stimulation have also revealed the importance of the site of application of the TENS electrodes. Pertovaara (1980) used a 'thermostimulator' to apply thermal stimuli either proximal or distal to TENS electrodes attached to the extensor surface of the forearm. The thermostimulator was composed of Peltier elements and had a built-in thermocouple connected to an oscilloscope for temperature measurements. The TENS treatment consisted of high frequency stimulation (100 Hz) delivered at an intensity of 35/45 mA (the authors did not specify the duration of application). Thermal pain threshold was elevated in only one of the six subjects used in the study when thermal pain threshold was measured distal to site of the 35 mA intensity TENS. However, the thermal pain threshold was significantly elevated in five out of six subjects (p < 0.02) when the thermal

stimuli were applied distal to the 45 mA intensity TENS. Interestingly, there were no significant increases in pain threshold when TENS was applied at 45 mA and thermal pain threshold measured at a proximal site. These results have therefore shown that a proximal site of TENS application coupled with a high current intensity produced an increase in pain threshold. In providing an explanation of the observed effects, the authors suggested that peripheral electrogenic blockade or fatigue of pain-mediating fibres was responsible for the elevation of pain threshold.

Sagers & Byrd (1983) used so-called 'radiant heat C Fibre Pain Threshold [CFPT]' to determine the analgesic effect of continuous 2 minute TENS hyperstimulation to the ho-ku acupuncture point (dorsum of hand in the angle of the first and second metacarpals; Chaitow 1983). A 250 watt 'dolorimeter' was used to apply radiant heat to the fifth distal phalanx and the time taken to produce an 'intense burning sensation' was measured. This type of painful sensation is mediated by the small diameter C (Group III) afferent fibres, hence the term CEPT. The application of TENS, even for this short period of time, resulted in a significant increase in CEPT (p < 0.05) in the experimental group compared to controls. These results indicate that TENS may modulate C fibre pain transmission and thus support the conclusion of Pertovaara (1980), i.e. TENS may produce a blockade of afferent nociceptive activity.

The face has also been used as site of application for thermal pain. Marchand et al (1991) applied thermal stimuli to the subjects' cheeks using a contact thermode. For this study, the TENS electrodes were placed over the maxillary branch of the trigeminal nerve to deliver electrical stimulation (125 μs, 100 Hz) for 25 minutes. Analysis of results showed that both during and after TENS, the thermal pain threshold was significantly increased (p = 0.002). In addition, the perceived intensity of noxious and near noxious heat stimuli during TENS was significantly reduced (p < 0.01). Interestingly, these researchers found that TENS had no effect on subjects' perception of light intensity assessed by the rating of visual stimuli from an incandescent bulb; the authors therefore concluded that TENS did not achieve hypoalgesia by a general distraction effect.

Eriksson et al (1985) designed a study to investigate whether TENS induced central changes in humans by examining thermal thresholds within (ipsilateral application) and outside (contralateral application) the innervation area of the stimulated nerve bundle. Thermal sensitivity was assessed over the thenar region during and post TENS applied over the median nerve (ipsilateral and contralateral). Thermal sensitivity was measured by asking subjects to indicate when they felt the temperature of the thermode stimulator change from hot to cold. Interestingly, similar effects were observed after 15 minutes' treatment with both conventional (80 Hz) and acupuncture-like (2 Hz) TENS. In addition, similar effects were seen for both contralateral and ipsilateral TENS application, therefore providing evidence that TENS-induced analgesia may be mediated by a central mechanism. This has important clinical implications with regard to electrode placement contralateral to the painful side, i.e. resulting in stimulation of the appropriate spinal segmental level.

In summary, these thermal pain studies have indicated the importance of both stimulation site and intensity. All the studies cited used either stimulation of a peripheral nerve or acupuncture point and (in most cases) the electrodes were positioned proximal to the site of experimental pain. The success of proximal application of TENS compared to a distal application adds strength to the hypothesis that TENS may indeed block or reduce the volume of incoming afferent nociceptive information. Although these studies have yielded interesting results, it is doubtful that the induced thermal pain approximates to clinical pain to any great extent, which therefore questions its validity as an experimental model.

Mechanical pain

Only three of the studies summarised in Table 5.2 used a mechanical pain model. Campbell & Taub (1973) investigated the effect of electrical stimulation on touch and pain threshold in response to needle stimuli delivered to the finger. Electrical

stimulation (100 Hz, 1 ms) at 10–12 V or 22 V was delivered to two electrodes positioned proximally on the finger. Results showed that electrical stimulation at 22 V significantly increased both touch ($p < 0.01$) and pain ($p < 0.001$) thresholds. In contrast, the 10–12 V intensity stimulation increased touch threshold only ($p < 0.5$).

Woolf (1979) applied mechanical pressure pain to the middle phalanx of the subject's finger. The apparatus consisted of a movable grip and a fixed restraining bar which allowed even distribution of mechanical stimulation. Values for threshold and tolerance pressure were taken. TENS (100 Hz, 0.25 ms, 10 ± 1 V) was applied for 30 minutes via two electrodes positioned over the ulnar nerve. This experiment found no significant changes in either pain threshold or tolerance following TENS application.

The only other study to date which has used mechanical pain as a model to investigate TENS analgesia was performed at the University of Ulster (Walsh et al 1995a). In this study, four TENS groups were compared with a control and placebo group. The TENS groups consisted of combinations of the following parameters: pulse frequency of 4 and 110 Hz, pulse duration of 50 and 200 µs. TENS was applied for three consecutive 5-minute periods via two electrodes attached to the skin directly over the course of the superficial radial nerve in the forearm. Mechanical pain threshold (MPT) measurements were taken from three standardised points in the first dorsal web space (this area of skin is innervated by the superficial radial nerve). A pressure algometer was mounted on a stand and a lever arm used to gradually lower the circular probe head (1.5 cm diameter) of the algometer to make contact with the skin at each of the three points to measure the pain threshold. At the distal point where control subjects recorded the most pain, repeated measures ANOVA (analysis of variance) found significant differences between groups ($p = 0.0101$), with the 110 Hz, 200 µs TENS group producing the greatest increase in pain threshold. This experiment is one of the few to investigate the effect of parameter combinations and should be viewed with the neurophysiological study also reported in the same paper.

Ischaemic pain

The submaximal effort tourniquet technique (SETT) is the most commonly used technique for induction of ischaemic pain. This technique involves the inflation of a sphygmomanometer cuff applied to the upper limb followed by a series of hand gripping exercises to induce ischaemic pain. Smith et al (1974) justify the use of the SETT as an experimental pain model as follows:

- the technique produces pain that resembles the duration and severity of many types of clinical pain
- it has been shown to have satisfactory test–retest reproducibility and sensitivity.

Walsh et al (1995c), Woolf (1979) and Roche et al (1984) used modified versions of the SETT to produce experimental ischaemic pain for the purposes of assessing TENS analgesia. In the study by Woolf (1979), the TENS electrodes were placed over the median and ulnar nerves proximal to the sphygmomanometer cuff. The stimulation (100 Hz, 0.25 ms, 10 ± 1 V) was applied for a period of 30 minutes before the SETT and during the test itself. After TENS, maximum tolerance time significantly increased (p < 0.001) and there was a subjective decrease in the assessment of pain (visual analogue scale (VAS) scores) compared to the control group.

Roche et al (1984) positioned the TENS electrodes over the radioulnar joint and cubital fossa to maximally stimulate the median and ulnar nerves. Based on this, it would appear that the electrodes were distal to the sphygmomanometer cuff. In contrast to the study by Woolf (1979), the analgesic effects of continuous (100 Hz, 1 ms) stimulation and train stimulation (5 Hz, 100 ms) were compared in this investigation. The stimulation intensity varied from a perceptible pricking sensation to a high non-noxious level (3.7–14.2 V) and was applied for 10 minutes prior to and during the SETT until tolerance was reported. Subjects who received the train stimulation mode at 'perceptible pricking sensation' intensities (3.7 V) showed significant increases in both pain threshold and pain tolerance (p < 0.01).

In contrast, the group which received high intensity (14.2 V) continuous TENS showed a significant increase in pain tolerance and endurance of ischaemia (p < 0.01), thus the latter type of stimulation appeared to be more effective in reducing experimental ischaemic pain. Although there were reductions in both visual analogue scales (VAS) and present pain intensity (PPI) scores in the TENS groups compared to controls, they were not significant.

In the most recent of the experimental ischaemic pain studies cited in Table 5.2, Walsh et al (1995c) compared the hypoalgesic effects of placebo, control, low (4 Hz) and high (110 Hz) frequency TENS (287 µs pulse duration). TENS was applied for 22 minutes over the ipsilateral Erb's point which overlies the brachial plexus. Results showed that low frequency TENS produced significantly greater hypoalgesia as assessed by VAS scores.

Delayed onset muscle soreness (DOMS)

Musculoskeletal pain has also been used as an experimental pain model. Delayed onset muscle soreness (DOMS) is the typical discomfort associated with unaccustomed exercise; it usually peaks 48 hours after the exercise. This type of experimental pain was used by Denegar et al (1989) to assess the analgesic effect of low frequency (2 Hz, 300 µs) TENS. DOMS was induced in the elbow flexors by repeated eccentric muscle work. TENS was applied 48 hours after the exercise session to four acupuncture points in the upper arm (TH14, LI11, LI13, LI14) for a 30-minute period at maximal tolerance intensity. Results showed that there was a significant decrease in perceived pain (p = 0.01; compared to pre-treatment value) following TENS treatment. There was no control group used in this study as the experimenters maintained that they could not justify inducing pain simply to document the normal course of DOMS; this lack of a control group obviously detracts from the significance of their findings.

An earlier study by Denegar & Huff (1988) used similar techniques to induce bilateral

DOMS in the elbow flexors. Subjects returned 48 hours after the initial pain-induction session and TENS was applied over the biceps brachii and brachialis muscles. Subjects received either high TENS (80 pps, ~90 μs) or low TENS (2 pps, 200 μs) stimulation for 30 minutes to the non-dominant or dominant arm. Results showed that there were no significant differences between high and low TENS or between treated and un-treated arms. Again, this study did not include a control group for the reasons already described above.

Jette (1987) compared the effects of high (85 Hz) and low (2 Hz) frequency TENS at both low and high intensity on exercise-induced muscle soreness in the wrist flexors. 48 hours after the pain-induction procedure, TENS was applied for 20 minutes (site of application was not given). Although results showed that TENS decreased the degree of muscle soreness to a greater extent during its application than after-wards, repeated measures ANOVA showed there was no significant treatment effect. Post hoc tests revealed significantly higher pain ratings both immediately and 20 minutes after TENS treatment. On the basis of these results, the author concluded that TENS effectiveness is independent of the frequency and intensity of stimulation.

There are a number of disadvantages asso-ciated with this model of experimental pain which make it an unsuitable experimental pain technique:

- the induced pain is not well characterised as a model of experimental pain
- the experimental procedure may be spread over a number of days, which makes subject compliance more difficult; for the purposes of selection of a suitable experimental model, this is a considerable disadvantage.

Cold-induced pain

Cold-induced experimental pain has been used to investigate the analgesic effects of TENS frequencies and pulse patterns respectively. The work of Johnson et al, who were based at the University of Newcastle upon Tyne, has made a noteworthy contribution to TENS research in this area. This group has published numerous well conducted studies on the effects of TENS on cold-induced pain, among others. In an early study by this group, Ashton et al (1984b) com-pared the effect of 8 Hz and 100 Hz TENS and needle acupuncture. The TENS (200 μs, 5.45 mA (8 Hz)/9.1 mA (100 Hz)) was applied to the ventral forearm, midway between the wrist and the elbow, for a 50-minute period. Acupuncture was administered to the wrist just above the 'Daling' point PC7. Ice pain threshold and toler-ance readings were taken for the purposes of analysis. There was an overall increase in both of these measurements in the 8 Hz TENS (not significant) and acupuncture groups (significant) compared with 100 Hz TENS or placebo groups. In the 8 Hz group, the increase in threshold and tolerance levels was accompanied by an increase in variance which, according to the authors, contributed to the non-significant differences observed in this group.

In a more recent study, Johnson et al (1989) compared the analgesic effect of 5 TENS fre-quencies (10–160 Hz) on cold-induced pain. The electrodes were placed over the median nerve, 3 cm above the proximal wrist crease. Stimula-tion (200 μs, 4.62–5.71 mA) was applied for 50 minutes. Interestingly, the results of this study conflict with the earlier study by the same group (Ashton et al 1984b). It was observed that TENS frequencies between 20 and 80 Hz produced the greatest increase in pain threshold. The com-bined TENS values (i.e. values for all the TENS groups taken as one group) showed a significant increase in ice pain threshold, compared with control or placebo values. In contrast, no signifi-cant differences in ice pain tolerance were found for TENS treatment.

There were some differences in experimental technique between the last two studies which may have contributed to the contrasting results. The position and size of electrodes used was not consistent between these studies; Johnson et al (1989) used smaller electrodes placed closer to the wrist. The electrode size is important, as the area and amount of stimulation delivered to the tissues will vary if inconsistent electrode sizes are used. Higher stimulation intensities were used in the earlier study to reach a 'strong but comfortable' level. In addition, Johnson et al (1989) suggest that the iced water rather than crushed ice used in the later study, may have reduced temperature variability from air pockets.

A further study by the same authors (Johnson et al 1991a) investigated the effects of five TENS pulse patterns, using the same experimental pain technique. The five types of output were burst, modulation, random (14–188 Hz), continuous and double-sized electrode continuous TENS. The electrode placement and duration of stimulation (200 µs, 80 Hz) were the same as in the previous study (Johnson et al 1989). Again, the combined TENS ice pain threshold values showed a significant increase compared to the control values ($p < 0.001$). All TENS pulse patterns used showed a significant increase in ice pain threshold over the experimental period with continuous mode showing the greatest increase. Ice pain tolerance was increased by all TENS modes with continuous mode showing the greatest increase again. Interestingly, the response was less in the continuous double-sized electrodes for both ice pain tolerance and threshold. These studies have emphasised that electrode position and size bear considerable relevance to the analgesic potential of TENS.

Johnson et al (1992) also compared the effectiveness of four different TENS modes on the model of cold pain described in their previous studies. The electrode placement sites and stimulation intensity used varied depending on the mode used; the duration of treatment was 30 minutes for all groups. Overall, the results showed variable effects of TENS upon pain threshold; continuous TENS mode increased pain threshold when electrical paraesthesia was achieved at the site of pain at both high (conventional TENS) or low (intense TENS) intensities. Burst mode TENS was effective when applied to a muscle mass myotomally-related to the painful site and only when the intensity was high enough to produce strong, forceful muscle contractions (i.e. acupuncture-like TENS). This paper has important clinical implications for choice of electrode placement sites and selection of appropriate stimulating modes.

The standardisation of temperature is a problem associated with the cold-induced pain technique which has been highlighted by the different results obtained in the studies conducted by Ashton et al (1984b) and Johnson et al (1989).

Electrical pain

Several studies have been conducted to examine the effect of auricular TENS upon experimental electrical pain (Johnson et al 1991b, Noling et al 1988, Oliveri et al 1986). Auricular TENS involves the application of electrical stimulation to acupuncture points on the external ear to relieve pain at distant sites. In the study by Johnson et al (1991b), a constant current stimulator was used to deliver square wave pulses (200 µs, 2 Hz) to the proximal interphalangeal joint and sensory and pain thresholds were measured. Auricular TENS (2.3 Hz pulse trains and 100 Hz within trains) was applied to three treatment points:

1. the 'wrist point', which was predicted to affect pain threshold
2. the 'autonomic point', which was predicted to affect autonomic function
3. the 'face point', which was used as a placebo point.

In addition, three autonomic parameters were recorded: blood pressure, skin temperature and heart rate. There were no significant differences found between combined TENS and control values for pain threshold. The pain threshold increased by over 30% during TENS in one third of subjects and by over 50% in four out of 18 subjects. No significant autonomic effects were observed following TENS.

Oliveri et al (1986) and Noling at al (1988) investigated the effect of auricular TENS upon electrical pain threshold measured at the wrist. Similar experimental procedures were used in both studies, the main difference being that the second study measured experimental pain threshold for 10 minutes post treatment compared with only an immediate post treatment measurement taken in the first study. Both studies contained control and placebo TENS groups as well as an active treatment group. In both studies, a significant increase in electrical pain threshold was observed only in the group which had auricular TENS applied to appropriate auricular acupuncture points; this effect was observed for the 10 minutes post treatment in Noling et al's study (1988).

Taylor et al (1993) reported significant differences between the effects of placebo and active auricular TENS on electrical threshold in the trigeminal nerve. In this study, three TENS groups were employed with frequencies of 5, 100 and 2000 Hz. Results showed that the 5 Hz and 100 Hz groups produced significantly greater hypoaesthesia (i.e. an increase in threshold) than the 2000 Hz group. As this review is directed towards cutaneous TENS application and not auricular TENS, these are the only auricular TENS studies that will be mentioned in this review.

Although electrical pain is a convenient method, Wolff (1978) points out that it produces a sensation referred to as 'discomfort' rather than 'pain' which limits its validity as an experimental model. A number of studies have been conducted to examine the analgesic effects of electrical stimulation upon experimental dental pain (Andersson & Holmgren 1978, Andersson et al 1977). These will not be included in this review as they are only of limited value to physiotherapy practice.

Experimental pain model criteria

This review has looked at a variety of experimental pain techniques. In order to select an appropriate technique a number of important criteria should be considered:

- The pain produced by the test should closely resemble clinical pain.
- There should be sufficient evidence that the test is reliable and reproducible.
- The test should provide a number of readings/values upon which efficacy can be quantitatively assessed.

Each experimental pain model has its own merits and disadvantages which have been identified in the sections in this chapter. Whatever pain model is chosen, it is important that the study has a comparative control/placebo group and is reproducible.

SUMMARY OF KEY POINTS

1. Stimulation parameter specific effects have been observed in several neurophysiological and experimental pain studies which are of clinical relevance.

2. There is now considerable evidence from neurophysiological studies that TENS may have a peripheral blocking effect on afferent nerve fibres; this effect appears to be associated only with high pulse frequencies.

REFERENCES

Andersson S A, Holmgren E 1978 Analgesic effects of peripheral conditioning stimulation-III: effect of high frequency stimulation; segmental mechanisms interacting with pain. Acupuncture and Electro-Therapeutics Research International Journal 3: 23–36

Andersson S A, Holmgren E, Roos A 1977 Analgesic effects of peripheral conditioning stimulation-II: importance of certain stimulation parameters. Acupuncture and Electro-Therapeutics Research International Journal 2(3,4): 237–246

Ashton H, Golding J F, Marsh V R, Thompson J W 1984a Effects of transcutaneous electrical nerve stimulation and aspirin on late somatosensory evoked potentials in normal subjects. Pain 18: 377–386

Ashton H, Ebenezer I, Golding J F, Thompson J W 1984b Effects of acupuncture and transcutaneous electrical nerve stimulation on cold-induced pain in normal subjects. Journal of Psychosomatic Research 28(4): 301–308

Campbell J N, Taub A 1973 Local analgesia from percutaneous electrical nerve stimulation. Archives of Neurology 28: 347–350

Chaitow L 1983 The acupuncture treatment of pain, 2nd edn. Thorsons Publishing Group, England

Chan C Y W, Tsang H 1987 Inhibition of the human flexion reflex by low intensity high frequency transcutaneous electrical nerve stimulation TENS has a gradual onset and offset. Pain 28: 239–253

Chung J M, Fang Z R, Hori Y, Lee K H, Willis W D 1984a Prolonged inhibition of primate spinothalamic tract cells by peripheral nerve stimulation. Pain 19: 259–275

Chung J M, Lee K H, Hori Y, Endo K, Willis W D 1984b Factors influencing peripheral nerve stimulation inhibition of primate spinothalamic tract cells. Pain 19: 277–293

Cox P D, Kramer J F, Hartsell H 1993 Effect of different TENS stimulus parameters on ulnar motor nerve conduction velocity. American Journal of Physical Medicine and Rehabilitation 72: 294–300

Denegar C R, Huff C B 1988 High and low frequency TENS in the treatment of induced musculoskeletal pain: a comparison study. Athletic Training 23(3): 235–237, 258

Denegar C R, Perrin D H, Rogol A D, Rutt R 1989 Influence of transcutaneous electrical nerve stimulation on pain, range of motion, and serum cortisol concentration in females experiencing delayed onset muscle soreness. Journal of Orthopaedic and Sports Physical Therapy 11(3): 100–103

Eriksson M B E, Rosén I, Sjölund B 1985 Thermal sensitivity in healthy subjects is decreased by a central mechanism after TNS. Pain 22: 235–242

Francini F, Maresca M, Procacci P, Zoppi M 1981 The effects of non-painful transcutaneous electrical nerve stimulation on cutaneous pain threshold and muscular reflexes in normal men and in subjects with chronic pain. Pain 11: 49–63

Francini F, Maresca M, Procacci P, Zoppi M 1982 Relationship between somatosensory evoked potential components and cutaneous pain threshold: effects of transcutaneous electrical nerve stimulation. In: Courjon J C, Mauguiere F, Revol M (eds) Clinical applications of evoked potentials in neurology. Raven Press, New York

Golding J F, Ashton A, Marsh R, Thompson J W 1986 Transcutaneous electrical nerve stimulation produces variable changes in somatosensory evoked potentials sensory perception and pain threshold: clinical implications for pain relief. Journal of Neurology Neurosurgery and Psychiatry 49: 1397–1406

Gracely R H 1991 Experimental pain methods. In: Max M, Portenoy R, Laska E (eds) Advances in pain research and therapy. Raven Press, New York, 18, pp. 33–47

Hui-Chan C, Levin M F 1993 Stretch reflex latencies in spastic hemiparetic subjects are prolonged after transcutaneous electrical nerve stimulation. Canadian Journal of Neurological Sciences 20(2): 97–106

Ignelzi R J, Nyquist J K 1976 Direct effect of electrical stimulation on peripheral nerve evoked activity: implications in pain relief. Journal of Neurosurgery 45: 159–165

Ignelzi R J, Nyquist J K 1979a Excitability changes in peripheral nerve fibers after repetitive electrical stimulation. Journal of Neurosurgery 51: 824–833

Ignelzi R J, Nyquist J K 1979b Observations on fast axoplasmic transport in peripheral nerve following repetitive electrical simulation. Pain 7: 313–320

Ignelzi R J, Nyquist J K, Tighe W J 1981 Repetitive electrical stimulation of peripheral nerve and spinal cord activity. Neurological Research 3(2): 195–209

Janko M, Trontelj J V 1980 Transcutaneous electrical nerve stimulation: a microneurographic and perceptual study. Pain 9: 219–230

Jette D U 1987 Effect of TENS frequency and intensity on exercise induced muscle soreness. Physical Therapy 67(5): 765

Johnson M I, Ashton C H, Bousfield D R, Thompson J W 1989 Analgesic effects of different frequencies of transcutaneous electrical nerve stimulation on cold-induced pain in normal subjects. Pain 39: 231–236

Johnson M I, Ashton C H, Bousfield D R, Thompson J W 1991a Analgesic effects of different pulse patterns of transcutaneous electrical nerve stimulation on cold-induced pain in normal subjects. Journal of Psychosomatic Research 35(2/3): 313–321

Johnson M I, Hajela V K, Ashton C H, Thompson J W 1991b The effects of auricular transcutaneous electrical nerve stimulation (TENS) on experimental pain threshold and autonomic function in healthy subjects. Pain 46: 337–342

Johnson M I, Ashton C H, Thompson J W 1992 Analgesic effects of acupuncture-like transcutaneous electrical nerve stimulation (TENS) on cold-induced pain (cold-pressor pain) in normal subjects. European Journal of Pain 13(4): 101–108

Katims J J, Ng L K Y 1985 Transcutaneous electrical stimulation TNS frequency dependent regional increases in rat brain metabolic activity. Acupuncture and Electro-Therapeutics Research International Journal 10(3): 223–224

Levin M F, Hui-Chan C 1993 Conventional and acupuncture-like transcutaneous electrical nerve stimulation excites similar afferent fibers. Archives of Physical Medicine and Rehabilitation 74: 54–60

Marchand S, Bushnell M C, Duncan G H 1991 Modulation of heat pain perception by high frequency transcutaneous electrical nerve stimulation (TENS). Clinical Journal of Pain 1: 122–129

Melzack R, Wall P D 1965 Pain mechanisms: a new theory. Science 150: 971–979

Noling L B, Clelland J A, Jackson J R, Knowles C J 1988 Effect of transcutaneous electrical nerve stimulation at auricular points on experimental cutaneous pain threshold. Physical Therapy 68: 328–332

Oliveri A C, Clelland J A, Jackson J, Knowles C 1986 Effects of auricular transcutaneous nerve stimulation on experimental pain threshold. Physical Therapy 66: 12–16

Pertovaara A 1980 Experimental pain and transcutaneous electrical nerve stimulation at high frequency. Applied Neurophysiology 43: 290–297

Procacci P, Zoppi M, Maresca M 1979 Experimental pain in man. Pain 6: 123–140

Roche P A, Gijsbers K, Belch J J F, Forbes C D 1984 Modification of induced ischaemic pain by transcutaneous electrical nerve stimulation. Pain 20: 45–52

Sagers M, Byrd K E 1983 Effects of TENS hyperstimulation on C fiber pain threshold. Physical Therapy 63(4): 750

Salar G, Iob I, Mingrino S 1980 Cortical evoked responses and transcutaneous electrotherapy. Neurology 30: 663–665

Sjölund B H 1985 Peripheral nerve stimulation suppression of C-fiber-evoked flexion reflex in rats. Journal of Neurosurgery 63: 612–616

Smith G M, Chiang H T, Kitz R J, Antoon A 1974 Acupuncture and experimentally induced ischemic pain. In: Bonica J J (ed) Advances in neurology. Raven Press, New York, pp. 827–832

Taylor D N, Katims J J, Lorenz K Y 1993 Sine-wave auricular TENS produces frequency-dependent hypesthesia in the trigeminal nerve. Clinical Journal of Pain 9(3): 216–219

Torebjörk H E, Hallin R G 1974 Excitation failure in thin nerve fiber structures and accompanying hypalgesia during repetitive electric skin stimulation. In: Bonica J J (ed) Advances in neurology. Raven Press, New York, pp. 733–735

Walmsley R P, Monga T N, Prouix M 1986 Effect of transcutaneous nerve stimulation on sensory nerve conduction velocity: a pilot project. Physiotherapy Practice 2: 117–120

Walsh D M, Foster N E, Baxter G D, Allen J M 1995a Transcutaneous electrical nerve stimulation (TENS): relevance of stimulation parameters to neurophysiological and hypoalgesic effects. American Journal of Physical Medicine and Rehabilitation 74(3): 199–206

Walsh D M, Greer K, Baxter G D 1995b Relevance of transcutaneous electrical nerve stimulation parameters to neurophysiological effects. Proceedings, 12th International Congress of the World Confederation for Physical Therapy, p. 576

Walsh D M, Liggett C, Baxter G D, Allen J M 1995c A double blind investigation of the hypoalgesic effects of transcutaneous electrical nerve stimulation. Pain 61(1): 39–45

Wolff B B 1977 The role of laboratory pain induction methods in the systematic study of human pain. Acupuncture and Electro-Therapeutics Research International Journal 2(3,4): 271–305

Wolff B B 1978 Behavioural measurement of human pain. In: Sternbach R A (ed) Psychology of pain. Raven Press, New York

Woolf C J 1979 Transcutaneous electrical nerve stimulation and the reaction to experimental pain in human subjects. Pain 7: 115–127

Worth R M, Ochs S 1976 The effect of repetitive electrical stimulation on axoplasmic transport. Neuroscience Abstracts 70(2): 50

CHAPTER CONTENTS

Introduction   83
  Clinical studies   83

Clinical studies on TENS   84
Dysmenorrhoea   84
Low back pain   86
Labour pain   89
Arthritis   91
  TENS modes comparison   92
Postoperative pain   95
  Other pain conditions   99

Summary of key points   100

6

Review of clinical studies on TENS

INTRODUCTION

Chapter 5 reviewed the range of laboratory studies that have been completed on TENS. We now focus on the studies that have been performed in the clinical setting. A similar format to Chapter 5 is adopted for this review; summary tables (Tables 6.1–6.5) provide relevant details of the studies under specific headings and the salient points of each study are discussed in more detail in the text. Inclusion of the entire range of clinical studies on TENS which have been conducted is beyond the scope of this chapter. Therefore only the following five common conditions are reviewed:

- dysmenorrhoea
- low back pain
- labour pain
- arthritis
- postoperative pain.

The chapter begins with a brief introduction to clinical research.

Clinical studies

Single case studies, cross-sectional studies and cohort studies are examples of types of study design used in clinical research. However, the most rigorous type of clinical study design is the randomised controlled trial (RCT). In this design, patients are allocated randomly to one of several treatment groups, one of which is a placebo/control group. Randomisation means that all patients have equal chances of being allocated to the treatment or control group. It is crucial to have a control group to monitor the natural course of the condition and thus provide an accurate comparative group for the treatment group(s). The inclusion of a placebo group allows the researcher to estimate the 'placebo response' to a specific treatment. In this review, the reader will note that a number of studies have included both control and placebo TENS groups. Indeed, some confusion exists regarding the differences between a placebo and control group in a clinical study; this can be easily clarified using TENS as an example. A placebo TENS group is one in which the TENS is applied in the same manner as the active TENS group, i.e. electrode placement site, instructions, etc., but the TENS unit has been rendered inactive. A control group is one in which only standard treatment is given, e.g. in postoperative pain studies the control group receives standard narcotic analgesia. Some authors incorrectly use the term control group when in fact placebo TENS has been applied.

In this chapter the reader will come across crossover designs in several of the reviewed studies. This study design involves all patients receiving each treatment in a specified sequence instead of being allocated to only one treatment group. Care must be taken to ensure that adequate time is allowed between each treatment so that there are no carry-over effects from one treatment to another. In addition, if placebo TENS is given first and then active TENS or vice versa, the patient may suspect which treatment was 'real' thus adding an element of bias to subjective pain scores.

The clinical trial is generally accepted as the only way of firmly establishing a cause–effect relationship between a given treatment and an observed outcome; however, the financial cost and lack of patient compliance are two examples of the problems associated with this type of study. Nevertheless, clinicians should not be discouraged from undertaking RCTs because such research can only serve to improve clinical practice. The reader is referred to a recent review by Ernst & Resch (1996) for further background to the clinical trial.

CLINICAL STUDIES ON TENS
Dysmenorrhoea

Dysmenorrhoea is lower abdominal pain experienced around the time of menstruation; primary dysmenorrhoea is defined as pain during menstruation for which there is no obvious cause, whereas secondary dysmenorrhoea is pain due to some underlying pathology (Beard & Pearce 1989). The basis of pain during menstruation is believed to be linked to the presence of prostaglandins in the menstrual fluid; prostaglandins cause hypercontractility of the myometrium (muscular layer of the wall of the uterus) which in turn causes uterine ischaemia. Successful pharmacological management of dysmenorrhoea involves the use of prostaglandin synthetase inhibitors; however, due to side-effects, some women cannot take these drugs. A non-pharmacological alternative would therefore be of considerable value in the management of dysmenorrhoea.

Studies investigating the effect of TENS on dysmenorrhoea have typically compared TENS with placebo TENS or an analgesic drug (see Table 6.1). Overall results have been favourable in terms of the amount of pain relief obtained. Kaplan et al (1994) obtained baseline pain scores from a group of sixty-one women during two menstrual cycles. Then TENS (100 Hz, 95 µs) was applied for an unspecified time during the next two cycles using a triangular electrode arrangement over an area corresponding to the T10, 11 and 12 dermatomes (the nerve roots which supply sensory fibres to the uterus). Analysis of pain scores after the two TENS cycles showed that 59% of patients had moderate pain relief, 31.2% had relief and 10% found no influence of TENS on their pain. Neighbors et al (1987) also reported significant ($p < 0.05$) analgesic results for one treatment with acupuncture-like TENS compared with a placebo sugar pill in their sample of 20 patients. TENS (1 Hz, 40 µs, 30 minutes) was applied bilaterally over four acupuncture points (B21, B29, ST36 and SP6).

Another group compared conventional and acupuncture-like TENS with a placebo group (the authors call this a control group even though

Table 6.1   Clinical studies on TENS (dysmenorrhoea)

Reference	Condition	n	Treatment	Electrodes	Results
Mannheimer & Whalen 1985	Dysmenorrhoea	27	1) Conventional TENS 125 Hz, 30 μs 2) Acupuncture-like TENS 2 Hz, 250 μs 3) Placebo TENS Duration = 30 min per Rx first, then used when pain returned	Groups 1 + 3 = 2 channels at level of umbilicus + ASIS Group 2 = bilateral SP6 + SP10	Sig dec pain and longer pain relief for conventional TENS vs placebo TENS
Neighbors et al 1987	Primary dysmenorrhoea	20	1) Placebo sugar pill 2) TENS 1 Hz, 40 μs, 30 min highest tolerable intensity	Bilateral B21, B29, ST36 and SP6	Sig pain relief in TENS group vs placebo group
Dawood & Ramos 1990	Primary dysmenorrhoea	32	1) TENS 100 Hz, 100 μs comfortable intensity 2) Placebo TENS Duration = first 8 hours then as needed 3) Ibuprofen 400 mg × 4/day	3 electrodes in Δ arrangement Positive = midline at T12 dermatome Two neg = lat to midline at T10–11 dermatome	Sig more pts did not need extra meds in TENS vs 2 and 3 groups. TENS sig delayed need for extra medication
Kaplan et al 1994	Primary dysmenorrhoea	61	TENS 100 Hz, 95 μs Duration = ?	3 electrodes in Δ arrangement Positive = midline at T12 dermatome Two neg = lat to midline at T10–11 dermatome	After TENS use: 59% pts = moderate relief, 31.2% pts = relief, 10% pts = no relief
Milsom et al 1994	Primary dysmenorrhoea	12	1) Naproxen 500 mg 2) TENS 70–100 Hz, 0.2 ms high intensity Duration = until pain relief	Lower abdomen and back	Both naproxen and TENS sig decrease pain Naproxen group – sig decrease all uterine activity parameters

Abbreviations:
ASIS = anterior superior iliac spine; **Cont** = continuous; **Inc** = increase; **Int** = intensity; **Sig** = significant.

placebo TENS was applied). Mannheimer & Whalen (1985) applied conventional and placebo TENS via a two-channel, criss-cross electrode arrangement at the level of the umbilicus and anterior superior iliac spine; bilateral SP6 and SP10 acupuncture points were used for the acupuncture-like TENS group. In this study, treatment time was kept constant at 30 minutes for all patients; patients were told to resume treatment when the pain returned throughout their menstrual cycle (i.e. home use of TENS was allowed). It appears that 2 Hz and 250 µs stimulation parameters were used for acupuncture-like TENS and 125 Hz and 30 µs were used for conventional TENS, although these details are not very clear in the text. Results showed that conventional TENS was significantly better than the placebo TENS for mean percentage pain relief ($p < 0.05$) and for the duration of pain relief (however, it should be noted that the level of significance was changed from $p < 0.05$ to $p < 0.1$ for the latter variable).

The three studies discussed above have demonstrated positive results for TENS analgesia, but how does TENS compare with common pharmacological interventions in dysmenorrhoea? The next two studies answer this very question. Dawood & Ramos (1990) compared TENS, placebo TENS and ibuprofen in a randomised four-way crossover study of 32 women suffering from primary dysmenorrhoea (the effectiveness of ibuprofen for relief of dysmenorrhoea is well established). The crossover design involved all women receiving each of the three types of treatment in a randomised fashion during four successive menstrual cycles: two TENS cycles and one cycle each for ibuprofen and placebo TENS. TENS electrodes were arranged in a manner similar to that used by Kaplan et al (1994), i.e. to stimulate the T10–12 dermatomes. The treatment time was considerably longer in this study; TENS (100 Hz, 100 µs) was applied continuously for the first 8 hours of the cycle and then used as required thereafter. The amounts of 'rescue medication' (i.e. ibuprofen) required during the TENS or placebo TENS cycles was also monitored. Results showed that a significantly greater number of patients who had TENS did not require 'rescue

medication' compared with the other two groups ($p < 0.01$); in addition, the use of TENS also significantly delayed the need for additional ibuprofen ($p < 0.05$).

The final study in this section directly compared one single dose of naproxen (500 mg) with TENS (0.2 ms, 70–100 Hz) over two menstrual cycles (Milsom et al 1994). This was another crossover study with all 12 patients receiving each treatment for one cycle. This study monitored pain scores and intrauterine pressure. TENS was applied over the lower abdomen and back and stimulation was repeated until pain relief was obtained. Both treatments significantly reduced pain but, interestingly, naproxen also significantly suppressed all uterine activity parameters ($p < 0.01$), e.g. resting pressure, active pressure, whereas TENS did not. As these results indicated that TENS analgesia was not related to changes in intrauterine pressure, the question of how TENS decreases pain in dysmenorrhoea remains. The authors discussed several theories and eventually suggested that TENS analgesia in dysmenorrhoea may be secondary to a reduction of myometrial ischaemia due to a local increase in blood flow or a decrease in oxygen consumption.

Low back pain

Low back pain (LBP) is one of the most common medical conditions to affect modern society. In addition to the pain and disability associated with this condition, the combined effect of lost working days and financial cost due to delayed accurate diagnosis, surgery and rehabilitation dictates that the development of an optimal treatment is a priority for health care resources. TENS has traditionally been regarded as one of the most popular conservative approaches to LBP. In contrast to the confirmed efficacy of TENS for dysmenorrhoea, studies on LBP have largely been negative. However, many flaws in methodology and treatment regime may have contributed to the negative findings in this area. In this section, eight studies have been selected which have compared TENS with placebo TENS, different modes of TENS and other therapeutic techniques (see Table 6.2).

Table 6.2 Clinical studies on TENS (low back pain [LBP])

Reference	Condition	n	Treatment	Electrodes	Results
Fox & Melzack 1976	Chronic LBP	12	1) TENS 60 Hz trains at 3 Hz train rate Intensity – painful level Duration = 10 min per point 2) Needle acupuncture 1 min/point	B24, B26 and B62 for both groups TENS – indifferent electrode placed at a distant site	No sig difference between groups for duration or amount of pain relief
Laitinen 1976	Sacrolumbalgia & ischialgia	100	1) Acupuncture 2) TENS 50 Hz, 1 ms Intensity – pricking sensation/numbness Duration both Rx = 20 min once a week for 2–10 Rxs	5 points used for both groups 2 points used bilaterally for each treatment	No sig difference between groups for pain relief
Melzack et al 1980	Chronic LBP	44	1) TENS 3 Hz Mildly painful intensity 2) Ice massage Duration both Rx = 30 min for 2 Rxs	B24, B26 and B62; indifferent electrode at back of knee	PRI – no sig difference between groups PPI – sig greater decrease in ice massage group
Melzack et al 1983	Acute & chronic LBP	41	1) TENS 4–8 Hz, tolerable intensity 2) Mechanical massage Duration both Rx – 30 min × 2/week for a max of 10 Rxs	Active = centre of pain Indifferent = lateral aspect of thigh	TENS – sig greater pain relief and sig improvement in SLR No sig difference between groups for range of flexion
Lehmann et al 1986	Chronic LBP	54 (–11)	1) Placebo TENS 2) TENS 60 Hz, 250 μs Subthreshold intensity ? Duration of 1 and 2 = 5/week for 3 weeks 3) Electroacupuncture 2–4 Hz, tolerable Intensity, ? duration, 2/week for 3 weeks	1 and 2 = centre of pain and related nerve trunk if significant leg pain 3 = variety of points	No sig difference between groups
Deyo et al 1990	Chronic LBP	145 (–20)	1) TENS and exercise 2) TENS only 3) Sham TENS and exercise 4) Sham TENS only Duration for all Rx = 45 min at least 3/day for 4 weeks	Initially over area of most severe pain, then moved as necessary	No sig difference between active and sham TENS TENS adds no benefit to exercise alone
Marchand et al 1993	Chronic LBP	42	1) TENS 100 Hz, 125 μs Intensity – clear but unpainful paraesthesia 2) Placebo TENS Duration = 30 min, 2/week for 10 weeks 3) Control	Optimal site determined for each pt	TENS – sig short term analgesia (immediately post Rx and 1 week after course of Rx finished) No significant differences between groups for long term effects (3 and 6 months after course of Rx finished)
Herman et al 1994	Acute LBP	58 (–17)	1) TENS/Codetron plus exercise 2) Placebo TENS/Codetron plus exercise Duration of 1 and 2 = 30 min/day, 5/week × 4 weeks	7 electrodes used. Pos = GV14 3 pairs neg bilateral at B23/24, B49/GB30 and B54	No sig difference between groups

Abbreviations: PPI = present pain index; **PRI** = pain rating index; **Sig** = significant; **SLR** = straight leg raise.
Note: the number in brackets in the 'n' column indicates the number of patients who did not complete the study.

Deyo et al published results of a randomised controlled clinical trial in 1990 which brought TENS into considerable disrepute in the USA. The impact of this study even caused some insurance companies to stop coverage of TENS therapy! Chronic LBP patients were recruited by newspaper advertisement and subsequently screened and interviewed; 145 LBP patients were recruited, 20 of whom later dropped out. Deyo et al compared four treatment groups in their study; these groups combined active or sham (placebo) TENS with or without a set of exercises. Patients received active/sham TENS at least three times a day for 45 minutes over 4 weeks. The active TENS group used conventional TENS (80–100 Hz) for the first 2 weeks, then tried acupuncture-like TENS (2–4 Hz) for an unspecified treatment time. Patients selected whichever mode they preferred for the remaining 2 weeks. Here lies the first major problem; as acupuncture-like TENS is believed to operate via endogenous opiate-mediated mechanisms, analgesia is typically longer in duration but has a longer onset latency (see Ch. 2). If the patients were only allowed to try this mode once and then had to make a quick decision, they may have missed out on potentially better analgesic effects with this mode. In addition, the authors state that a modulated frequency output was used for both TENS modes; this was a strange choice, particularly for a clinical trial, because the efficacy of this type of output has not been thoroughly investigated. Patients also received heat treatment when they attended the clinic and were loaned electric heating pads for home use. The introduction of this additional therapy may be seen as a confounding variable with respect to the results obtained. Four categories of outcome measures were used for analysis: functional status, pain ratings, physical measures and use of medical services. Results showed no significant differences in any outcome measure between the active and sham TENS groups and therefore the authors concluded that TENS may be no better than placebo and that TENS and exercise was no better than TENS alone. This RCT had an impressive number of patients and was very thorough in measurement of a range of treatment outcomes, but due to oversights in the treatment regime the results have to be interpreted cautiously.

Marchand et al (1993) also used a group of chronic LBP patients to examine whether TENS analgesia was purely a placebo effect. Active TENS (100 Hz, 125 µs) was compared with placebo TENS and a group of controls (no treatment) was also included. The short and long term analgesic effects of each treatment were monitored by use of VAS. Patients were treated for a 30-minute period, twice a week for 10 weeks. In this study, an evaluation was made to determine optimal electrode positioning for each patient before treatment commenced (this is an important procedure which should be adopted in all clinical trials in this area). Results showed that TENS was significantly better than placebo TENS in reducing pain intensity ($p = 0.05$) but not unpleasantness in the short term, i.e. immediately post treatment and 1 week after the course of treatment finished. There was also a significant additive/cumulative treatment effect for TENS which was not evident for placebo TENS. However, there were no significant differences between active and placebo TENS for pain intensity 3 and 6 months post treatment. This was a well conducted study with excellent attention to selection of appropriate treatment regime.

A more recent study by Herman et al (1994) compared active and placebo TENS plus a standard exercise programme for acute LBP over a 4-week period. In this study, the TENS used was a specific type called Codetron which randomly switches stimulation among six electrode sites every 10 seconds. Three pairs of negative electrodes were applied bilaterally at three levels over acupuncture points (B23/24, B49/GB30, B54) and the positive electrode was placed at GV14. The Codetron treatment consisted of 15 minutes high frequency TENS (200 Hz) followed by 15 minutes acupuncture-like TENS (4 Hz); treatment was given 5 days a week for 4 weeks. Although both treatment groups improved significantly during the 4-week programme, no additional benefits were observed for the TENS/Codetron group in terms of disability, pain, muscle strength and return to work. The authors therefore agreed with Deyo et al (1990), saying that TENS combined with exercise did not result in better outcomes than exercise alone.

The next three studies compared TENS with either acupuncture or electroacupuncture for chronic LBP. Lehmann et al's (1986) study failed to show any significant differences between active TENS, placebo TENS and electroacupuncture; however, the electroacupuncture group consistently showed greater improvements. In the active and placebo TENS groups, treatment was applied over the centre of pain and over a related nerve trunk if there was significant leg pain. Electroacupuncture was delivered via a needle to a variety of points. It caused some concern to read that patients in the electroacupuncture group often had 'other aches and pains' treated concomitant with the LBP treatment; perhaps this may have contributed to the better overall performance in this group. Fox & Melzack (1976) failed to demonstrate significant differences between needle acupuncture and TENS (60 Hz, train rate 3 Hz) for amount or duration of pain relief. Each treatment was applied over the same acupuncture points; all 12 subjects received two acupuncture and two TENS treatments at weekly intervals. In the same year, Laitinen (1976), using a larger group of patients (n = 100) suffering from chronic sacrolumbalgia and ischialgia, also failed to demonstrate significant differences between needle acupuncture and TENS (50 Hz, 1 ms) applied over a set of acupuncture points. It would appear from these two studies that TENS and needle acupuncture may be equally effective.

Mechanical massage and ice massage have also been used as comparative treatments for TENS in the management of LBP. Melzack et al (1983) compared TENS applied to the area of back pain with mechanical massage applied via four suction cups from an apparatus that produced changes in pressure. Both treatments were given for 30 minutes, twice a week for a maximum of 10 treatments. All patients also received standard exercises for LBP. Results from McGill Pain Questionnaire (MPQ) data showed that TENS was more effective for pain relief (p < 0.001); additionally, there was a significant increase in straight leg raise on both sides but no significant increase in range of lumbar flexion in the TENS group.

Melzack et al (1980) also compared ice massage and TENS for chronic LBP: treatment was applied over the same acupuncture points used in the Fox & Melzack study (1976). A group of 44 chronic LBP patients received two treatments of each technique at intervals of 1–2 weeks. There was a significantly greater decrease (p < 0.02) in PPI scores (taken from McGill Pain Questionnaire (MPQ); see Ch. 7) in the ice massage group compared with the TENS when the two treatments were compared for all patients; no significant differences were observed for pain rating index (PRI) scores.

Several discrepancies in the general methodology and TENS treatment regime may have contributed to the overall mixed results in the selected LBP studies. The next section focuses again on LBP, but in this case it is acute LBP combined with abdominal pain, both of which are experienced in labour.

Labour pain

The intensity and area of pain varies considerably during the different stages of labour (see Ch. 7, Fig. 7.9). During the first stage of labour, the dilatation of the cervix and contractions of the uterus cause pain in the abdomen and back; in late first stage, the pain tends to be mainly suprapubic. In the second stage, distension of the perineum and pressure on pelvic organs are additional sources of pain. There are two standard electrode placement sites for labour pain. Pairs of electrodes are placed paravertebrally, at the level of T10–L1 and at S2–S4 level, because these are the spinal segments which ultimately receive nociceptive information from the uterus, cervix and perineal structures. The upper pair of electrodes therefore targets pain during the first stage of labour while the lower is directed at second stage pain. In some cases, suprapubic electrodes have also been used; however, in those studies which have reported success with TENS, it is primarily relief of LBP with little or no effect on abdominal/suprapubic pain. Table 6.3 summarises the studies reviewed in this section.

Table 6.3 Clinical studies on TENS (labour pain)

Reference	Condition	n	Treatment	Electrodes	Results
Augustinsson et al 1977	Labour pain	147	TENS 0.25 ms, frequency chosen by each pt Hand held switch for different intensity levels	Two channels 1) T10–L1 2) S2–S4	Pain relief: 44% = very good/good 44% = moderate 12% = no effect
Bundsen et al 1981	Labour pain	566	1) TENS 2) Control	Refer to Augustinsson et al 1977	TENS group – 40% had good relief from back pain Control group – 20% had good relief from back pain TENS had a specific effect on back pain and not on suprapubic pain
Nesheim 1981	Labour pain	71	1) TENS 100 Hz, 0.25 ms Intensity highest level that felt comfortable Switch for stronger stimulation 2) Placebo TENS	Two channels 1) T10–L1 2) S2–S4	No sig difference between groups for pain relief or request for additional analgesia
Harrison et al 1986	Labour pain	150	1) TENS 80–100 Hz, 60–80 μs Burst mode available 2) Placebo TENS	Two channels 1) T10–L1 2) S2–S4	No sig difference between groups for pain relief Evident consumer satisfaction
Harrison et al 1987	Labour pain	170	1) TENS 80–100 Hz, 60–80 μs Burst mode available 2) Entonox 3) Pethidine and promazine 4) Lumbar epidural	Two channels 1) T10–L1 2) S2–S4	Complete relief – 88% epidural pts Partial relief – 90% entonox pts, 96% TENS pts & 54% pethidine and promazine pts Evident consumer satisfaction
Thomas et al 1988	Labour pain	280	1) Placebo TENS 2) TENS ? parameters	Two channels 1) T10–L1 2) S2–S4	No sig difference between groups for pain relief or request for additional analgesia
Bortoluzzi et al 1989	Labour pain	60	1) TENS approx 100 Hz, 100 μs Boost control for increasing current 2) Control	Two channels 1) T10–L1 2) S2–S4 Suprapubic electrodes also available	Sig less pethidine used in TENS group. When pts acted as their own controls, sig pain relief in TENS group High consumer satisfaction

Abbreviations:
Sig = significant.

Obstetric TENS studies date back to the 1970s; an early study by Augustinsson et al (1977; not in summary table) evaluated the effect of TENS in a sample of 147 women by feedback from questionnaires. In addition to TENS, extra pain relief was given on request to all patients. Results showed that 44% of patients reported very good/good pain relief with TENS, 44% reported moderate relief while 10% reported no effect. Bundsen et al (1982) also used a questionnaire to evaluate the effect of conventional analgesia in 544 parturients within 2 hours of delivery. Pain relief was given according to patients' wishes; interestingly, it was reported that TENS and/or diazepam were given to less than 10% of this study sample and almost never to those arriving in the labour ward in late stages of labour.

A common feature of obstetric TENS studies is the assessment of treatment efficacy by determining the amount of additional pain relief that is requested by patients. Bortoluzzi (1989) reported that significantly less pethidine was used in a TENS group (approximately 100 Hz and 100 μs) compared to a control group in his sample of 60 parturients. Additionally, there was a significant decrease in pain perception when TENS was switched on compared to when it was switched off (i.e. patients acted as their own controls). This study also reported a high level of satisfaction among patients: 100% of the TENS group said they would use it again for future deliveries.

In contrast, another controlled study by Bundsen et al (1981) compared 283 parturients who used TENS with the same number of matched controls. Questionnaire results indicated that in the early first stage, 40% of the TENS patients experienced good relief of back pain compared with 20% of the control patients. However, relatively few women in either group experienced good relief of abdominal pain .

The following three studies have directly compared active and placebo TENS for labour pain. Thomas et al (1988), in their sample of 280 patients, neglected to specify the stimulation parameters used. The results showed no differences between groups for other analgesia required or pain relief. Nesheim (1981) similarly reported no

differences between TENS (100 Hz, 0.25 ms) and placebo TENS for pain relief or amount of analgesics used. Harrison et al (1986) commented on evident consumer satisfaction with obstetric TENS, although this group also found no differences between active and placebo TENS in a group of 150 parturients. A further study by Harrison et al (1987) compared the effectiveness of 170 patients' initial choice of analgesia: TENS, Entonox, lumbar epidural, pethidine and promazine. Overall, 88% of patients who chose epidural reported complete pain relief; partial pain relief was reported by 90% of Entonox patients, 96% of TENS patients and 54% of pethidine and promazine patients. Consumer satisfaction of TENS patients was again reported in this study, with 60% of the TENS group stating that they would use TENS again; however, this satisfaction should be compared with the relatively higher number of epidural patients (88%) who said they would use this method of analgesia again.

Reports of artefacts in foetal heart rate traces when obstetric TENS was used simultaneously with internal monitoring caused obvious concern in the early years (Augustinsson et al 1977, Bundsen et al 1981); it has subsequently been reported that this interference can be effectively suppressed by using a filter (Bundsen & Ericson 1982). More importantly, no adverse effects have been observed in either mother or foetus in several studies (Bundsen & Ericson 1982, Harrison et al 1986). The overall impression from the eight studies reviewed is that despite consumer satisfaction, obstetric TENS fails to produce analgesia equivalent to conventional labour analgesia, specifically epidural analgesia. However, it would appear that TENS should continue to be offered as a method of analgesia in view of the following advantages associated with TENS:

- the parturient remains alert during labour and has an active role in the use of TENS
- there are no side-effects
- it is non-invasive.

Arthritis

In contrast to the conditions discussed above, the application of TENS for arthritic pain is more complex because of possible multijoint involvement. Even if TENS is recommended for home use, several consecutive electrode placement sites may have to be used in order to provide satisfactory relief.

Several studies have investigated the effectiveness of TENS for both osteoarthritis (OA) and rheumatoid arthritis (RA); the majority of studies utilise a crossover design to compare active and placebo TENS (see Table 6.4).

Three studies were conducted in the early 1980s which compared active and placebo TENS for OA knee pain. Lewis et al (1984) prepared patients for their crossover trial by using a pre-treatment 'washout' week during which paracetamol was the only medication used. After this baseline period, the 30 patients self-administered active TENS (70 Hz) and placebo TENS (3 weeks each treatment). Patients applied TENS for 30–60 minutes three times daily over classical acupuncture points around the knee. There was a significantly longer duration of relief after the active treatment (p < 0.01) and both active and placebo treatment provided more pain relief than paracetamol alone (p < 0.005). Overall, there was very little difference between the treatment response rate (46%) and the placebo response rate (43%). In another study on osteoarthritic knees, Smith et al (1983) showed a better TENS treatment response rate – 66.7% of TENS patients reported significant pain relief compared to 26.7% of the placebo TENS patients, although the differences between groups was not significant. In contrast to Lewis et al's study (1984), treatment in this study was given by a clinician.

The final study comparing active and placebo TENS was conducted by Taylor et al (1981); this group reported a significant difference between self-administered active TENS (parameters not specified) and placebo TENS for subjective pain score (p = 0.03) and medication score (p = 0.06) in a crossover study of 12 patients. However, no differences were noted for ambulation score or verbal pain score. It was interesting to note that in this study, subjects were told to self-administer TENS for 30-minute periods as required whereas in the latter two studies specific time periods were used.

Codetron TENS (previously discussed in LBP section) was compared with placebo Codetron in a group of 56 OA patients by Fargas-Babjak et al (1992). A range of acupuncture points was used for stimulation for 30 minutes twice daily over 6 weeks. The first two treatments were applied in a clinic and the remainder were self-administered at home. Analysis of a range of measurable outcomes including functional status, range of movement and pain only showed significantly more pain relief in the active Codetron TENS group compared to the placebo Codetron TENS (p < 0.02).

TENS modes comparison

The next group of studies which will be discussed compared the effectiveness of different TENS modes on both RA and OA pain. The first of these was conducted back in 1979 by Mannheimer & Carlsson on a group of 20 RA patients with severe wrist pain. All patients were treated for a 10-minute time period with all three modes of TENS in a random order: 70 Hz high frequency TENS, 3 Hz low frequency TENS and a train stimulation with 70 Hz internal frequency (repetition rate of 3 Hz). The duration of time between each treatment is unclear therefore it cannot be established if there was sufficient 'washout' time between treatments. Electrodes were placed proximal to the wrist on the volar and dorsal surface. Results showed that high frequency 70 Hz TENS and the train stimulation mode gave comparable levels of analgesia, while analgesia with the low frequency 3 Hz TENS was considerably less. The treatment time of 10 minutes was relatively short compared to the 30–60 minutes cited in the majority of other studies. As discussed in Chapter 2, acupuncture-like TENS analgesia involves opioid release and thus has a relatively longer onset latency; the treatment time in this study may not have been sufficient to achieve analgesia through the DPSS.

Langley et al (1984) used a similar electrode placement site in their study of 33 RA patients with chronic hand involvement. A crossover design was used to compare placebo TENS, high frequency TENS (0.2 ms, 100 Hz) and acupunc-

Table 6.4 Clinical studies on TENS (Rheumatoid arthritis and osteoarthritis)

Reference	Condition	n	Treatment	Electrodes	Results
Mannheimer & Carlsson 1979	RA wrist pain	20	1) TENS 70 Hz 2) TENS 3 Hz 3) Train stimulation 70 Hz internal freq 80 ms duration, 3 Hz repetition rate Int immediately below pain Duration all groups = 10 min	2 electrodes prox to wrist on volar and dorsal aspect	Comparable analgesia in 1 and 3, 2 much lower Average duration of pain relief: 1 = 18.2 hours 2 = 4 hours 3 = 15.2 hours
Taylor et al 1981	OA knee	12 (−2)	1) TENS (parameters not specified) 2) Placebo TENS Comfortable firm tingling sensation Duration of 1 and 2 = 30 min as required over 4 weeks	4 electrodes on anterior, posterior, medial and lateral aspects of knee	TENS sig better than placebo TENS for subjective pain score and medication score. No sig diff for ambulation or verbal pain score
Smith et al 1983	OA knee	32 (−2)	1) TENS 32–50 Hz, comfortable tingling 2) Placebo TENS Duration of 1 and 2 = 20 min/day × 8 Rxs over 4 weeks	4 electrodes on most tender points around the knee, usually acupuncture points	TENS group – 66.7% had significant pain relief Placebo group – 26.7% had significant pain relief
Langley et al 1984	RA & chronic hand pain	33	1) Placebo TENS 2) High freq TENS 0.2 ms, 100 Hz 3) Acupuncture-like TENS 2 Hz train 100 Hz internal freq 70 ms duration Highest tolerable intensity Duration all groups = 20 min	2 electrodes prox to wrist on volar and dorsal aspect	All 3 groups equally effective for analgesia
Lewis et al 1984	OA knee	30 (−2)	1) TENS 70 Hz 2) Placebo TENS Duration of 1 and 2 = 30 to 60 min/day 3 /day for 3 weeks	4 electrodes placed around knee at classical acupuncture points	43% response rate to placebo, 46% response rate to TENS Sig longer duration of relief after TENS Both 1 and 2 sig better than paracetamol
Bruce et al 1988	RA	8	1) TENS only 2) CBM only 3) CBM, CBM and TENS 4) TENS, CBM and TENS CBM approx 1.5 hours duration TENS approx 70 Hz, comfortable int producing paraesthesia Approx 20 min treatments	2 electrodes prox to wrist on volar and dorsal aspect	Combined TENS/CBM treatment may be effective, particularly when TENS applied first
Jensen et al 1991	OA knee	20	1) Low freq TENS 2 Hz trains 2) High freq TENS 80 Hz, 150 µs Max non-painful intensity Duration of 1 and 2 = 30 min daily × 5 days	Channel 1 = ST36/GB34 and Sp10 Channel 2 = Sp9 and ST34	No sig difference in pain level reported by the groups in any of 3 weeks, nor rest pain or consumption of analgesics/NSAIDs
Fargas-Babjak et al 1992	OA knee & hip	56 (−19)	1) CODETRON TENS 1 ms, 4 Hz train rate 200 Hz burst frequency 2) Placebo CODETRON duration of 1 and 2 = 30 min × 2/day × 6 weeks	7 electrodes used over acupuncture points: UB30, UB60, ST36, Sp9, GB34 GV14, LI4, Ah Chi and extra points	CODETRON sig more pain relief than placebo group

Table 6.4 (contd)

Reference	Condition	n	Treatment	Electrodes	Results
Grimmer 1992	OA knee	60	1) High rate TENS 80 Hz Strong tolerable, tingling paraesthesia 2) Strong burst mode TENS 3 Hz trains of 7 80 Hz pulses, strong tolerable tingling with visible muscle contraction Duration of 1 and 2 = 30 min 3) Placebo TENS	4 electrodes on Sp9, GB33, UB40 and Sp10	Sig greater decrease in knee circumference for 2 vs 1 Sig difference in length of pain relief, length of stiffness relief and range of movement for 2 vs 3 Sig difference in immediate stiffness relief and length of stiffness relief for 1 vs 3
Lewis et al 1994	OA knee	36 (−10)	1) Naproxen and placebo TENS 2) TENS & placebo naproxen 3) Placebo TENS and placebo naproxen TENS 70 Hz, 100 µs, 30–60 min × 3/day Highest comfortable amplitude Naproxen – 2 × 250 mg twice daily All treatments = 3 weeks	Sp9, Sp10, ST34 and ST35	No sig difference between groups

Abbreviations:
CBM = cognitive behaviour modification; **Prox** = proximal; **Sig** = significant.
Note: the number in brackets in the 'n' column indicates the number of patients who did not complete the study.

ture-like TENS (2 Hz train, 100 Hz internal frequency). Each treatment was given for 20 minutes at the highest intensity that could be tolerated. All three groups were found to be equally effective for improvements in rest pain, joint tenderness, grip strength and grip pain.

Both Grimmer (1992) and Jensen et al (1991) used four acupuncture points around the knee for comparison of high frequency TENS and burst mode/pulse train TENS in the treatment of OA of the knee. Jensen et al's study could not clearly demonstrate a difference between TENS groups for rest pain, pain relief or consumption of medication. However, Grimmer reported a number of significant differences between groups: burst mode TENS produced a significantly greater length of pain relief (p = 0.014), length of stiffness relief (p = 0.005) and change in range of movement (p = 0.03) than placebo TENS. Burst mode also produced a greater decrease in the circumference of the knee (p = 0.04) compared with high rate TENS. High rate TENS produced a greater length of stiffness relief (p = 0.004) compared with placebo TENS. Overall it would appear from this study that the burst mode of TENS was more effective at least compared to placebo TENS.

TENS has also been compared with conventional drug management of OA. In a recent study, Lewis et al (1994) reported no significant difference in a crossover trial which compared three treatment combinations:

- TENS plus placebo naproxen
- naproxen and placebo TENS
- placebo TENS and placebo naproxen.

All patients received each of the three combinations for a 3-week period. Results showed no significant difference between the three treatments.

The final study in this section was an interesting pilot study by Bruce et al (1988) who compared cognitive behaviour modification (CBM) and TENS for a small group of RA patients (n = 8). Patients were allocated to four groups (n = 2 each group): TENS only; CBM only; TENS combination which received TENS followed by a combination of CBM and TENS; and, finally, a CBM combination which received CBM followed by a combination of CBM and TENS. CBM included relaxation training and cognitive coping techniques. Grip strength, VAS, MPQ and joint evaluation were used as outcome variables. Results showed that the TENS combination group improved for all the self-reported pain scores. However, as the number of subjects in each group was very small (n = 2), it is difficult to draw conclusions from this study. Nevertheless, the idea of a cognitive behavioural/TENS approach to RA management certainly warrants further investigation.

Postoperative pain

Postoperative pain is acute, localised and usually lasts up to 72 hours. The relief of postoperative pain appears to be one of the most successful applications of TENS. Routine postoperative medication typically involves administration of opioids which have a number of unwanted side-effects (e.g. nausea, sedation, respiratory depression), therefore an uncomplicated alternative would be welcome. In most clinics, if TENS is used it is offered as an adjunct to routine medication rather than as a sole option. The pain-relieving effects of TENS may also indirectly affect postoperative lung function. The sooner a patient is ambulant post surgery, the more effectively she will cough and thereby remove unwanted secretions and reduce the risk of infection and atelectasis.

The success of postoperative TENS in clinical studies is usually assessed by the following measures:

- lung function tests, e.g. forced vital capacity (FVC), forced expiratory volume in 1 second (FEV_1) and peak expiratory flow rate (PEFR)
- pain relief at rest, while mobilising, during coughing
- requests for other pain medication
- length of stay in recovery room and in hospital.

The majority of studies which are discussed in this section describe similar electrode placement sites, i.e. the sterile TENS electrodes are typically positioned on either side of the surgical incision. A second pair of electrodes is sometimes placed over the thoracic spinal nerves which supply the dermatomes in the painful area (see Table 6.5).

In a recent study, Forster et al (1994) compared active TENS, placebo TENS and control treatments following coronary artery bypass graft (CABG) surgery. TENS was applied continuously for 48 hours via two pairs of electrodes placed either side of the incision and either side of T1–T5 spinous processes. A total of six measurements were used for analysis. The only significant finding was that rest pain was significantly lower in the TENS group compared with controls ($p < 0.04$). The other measurements which showed no significant differences were pain with cough, intake of narcotic medication, FVC, FEV_1 and PEFR. The authors reported no difference between active and placebo TENS, thus suggesting that TENS was not a useful adjunct to narcotic medications following CABG.

In contrast, Bayindir et al (1991) reported success with a 180 minute application of TENS following cardiac surgery. Pain score results were compared with a placebo TENS group. At the end of 180-minutes, 80% of the placebo group had severe chest pain and needed narcotics; at the same time point, 79% of TENS patients were completely free of resting chest pain. One of the main differences in TENS regime between this study and Forster et al's (1994) was the type of TENS mode. This study used burst TENS (burst mode: 10 pulses per burst, 2 bursts per second, 50–60 µs) whereas the latter used 287 Hz and 60 µs (i.e. more conventional TENS parameters). This difference in analgesia may be due to the role of opioids in low frequency TENS as discussed in Chapter 2.

A range of pulmonary function tests, narcotic requirements and pain scores were used as assessment measures for post thoracotomy pain relief in studies by Ho et al (1987) and Warfield et al (1985). Both of these studies failed to give specific details of the TENS parameters used. The parameters were set for each individual patient in Ho et al's study whereas Warfield et al only gave the parameter ranges available on the machine used. Two different treatment regimes were used in these two studies; Ho et al gave six 15-minute treatments over the first 3 postoperative days while Warfield et al's patients received continuous treatment for 48 hours. The lack of parameter details makes it difficult to draw conclusions from both studies, despite reports of significantly lower pain scores ($p = 0.014$) in the first 24 hours in the TENS group compared to placebo TENS (Warfield et al 1985) and a significant decrease in post versus pre TENS pain scores ($p < 0.001$; Ho et al 1987).

The site of the surgical incision has direct relevance to secondary pulmonary complications. The studies already mentioned have involved intrathoracic surgery which involves access via the rib cage. Surgical procedures which require an incision lower down (i.e. a midline or paramedian incision), can result in pulmonary complications due to ineffective coughing or deep breathing directly associated with abdominal musculature incisional pain. The following two studies assessed the efficacy of postoperative TENS in cholecystectomy patients in which the incisions were right upper paramedian (Sim 1991) and midline (Laitinen & Nuutinen 1991). Laitinen & Nuutinen (1991) allocated patients to one of four groups: control; an intravenous bolus of 25 mg indomethacin (non-steroidal anti-inflammatory drug; NSAID) followed by a continuous infusion of 5 mg of indomethacin in 1 hour; low frequency (2 Hz) TENS plus indomethacin as described; high frequency (100 Hz) TENS plus indomethacin as described. TENS was applied for 16 hours via two pairs of electrodes placed either side of the incision. Analysis of amount of rescue narcotics required showed no significant differences between the four groups.

During a 48-hour period, Sim (1991) compared the analgesic effectiveness of a control group who received a regimen of intramuscular papaveretum (an opiate analgesic) and a group which received TENS and supplementary intramuscular papaveretum. In contrast to the previous study, two electrodes were placed on both sides of the incision and a further two paravertebrally at the level of T7–T10. There was no significant

Table 6.5 Clinical studies on TENS (Postoperative)

Reference	Surgery	n	Treatment	Electrodes	Results
Issenman et al 1985	Spinal fusion	20	1) TENS Freq and pulse duration pre-set at mid range Comfortable int Duration = continuous 24 hour stimulation 2) Age- and sex-matched controls	2 electrodes placed 1.5 cm either side of incision and 2 electrodes placed either side of graft site incision	TENS pts received lower doses of pain medication
Warfield et al 1985	Thoracotomy	24	1) TENS ? parameters 2) Placebo TENS Duration = 48 hours	Electrodes placed 2 cm away from suture line	Sig lower pain scores in TENS group on day 1, no sig difference on day 2. TENS pts tolerated chest physio sig better on both days. Sig shorter stay in recovery room for TENS pts. No sig diff between groups for narcotic requirements or for nausea
Arvidsson & Eriksson 1986	Knee sx	15	1) Placebo TENS 2) TENS 100 Hz, 160 µs (as an average) Comfortable intensity Duration of 1 and 2 = 15 to 20 minutes 3) Epidural injection of local anaesthetic	2 electrodes placed med and lat to knee 2 electrodes placed at L3–L4 level	Epidural produced both the best pain relief and increase in quadriceps contraction, active TENS was next best while placebo TENS had no beneficial effect on either pain or contraction ability
Ho et al 1987	Thoracotomy	15	TENS intensity, frequency and duration set for each pt to give most comfort Duration = 6 × 15 min treatments over first 3 postop days.	2 electrodes placed diagonally across most painful part of thoracotomy wound	Sig decrease between pre and post TENS pain scores Sig higher FVC and FEV_1 after TENS
McCallum et al 1988	Lumbar laminectomy	20	1) TENS 70 Hz, 180 µs, comfortable int 2) Placebo TENS Duration 1 and 2 = 24 hours	2 electrodes placed parallel to incision 2 more placed at either end, i.e. at 90°	No sig diff between groups for no. of demands for patient-controlled analgesia
Bayindir et al 1991	Cardiac sx	89	1) TENS burst mode: 10 pulses/burst 2 bursts/sec, 50–60 µs Intensity inc until sensation felt on chest wall 2) Placebo TENS Duration of 1 and 2 = 180 min	2 electrodes on either side of sternotomy incision over area of max pain	After 180 minutes: 79% of TENS group = free of resting chest pain 80% of placebo group = severe chest pain and needed narcotics
Laitinen & Nuutinen 1991	Cholecystectomy	60	1) Control 2) Indomethacin 3) 2 Hz TENS & Indomethacin 4) 100 Hz TENS & Indomethacin Int and pulse duration adjusted to give max Int tol without unpleasant sensations Duration of TENS –16 hours	2 pairs placed either side of incision 1 pair at rostral end, other at caudal end	No sig difference between groups in amount of opiate required

Table 6.5 (contd)

Reference	Surgery	n	Treatment	Electrodes	Results
Sim 1991	Cholecystectomy	30	1) Control 2) TENS & supplementary intramuscular papaveretum Int, freq & pulse duration adjusted to give max comfort, continuous/intermittent use Duration = 48 hours	2 electrodes placed either side of incision 2 electrodes placed at level of T7–T10	TENS sig less rest and deep breathing pain on day 2 TENS sig less cough pain on day 5
Forster et al 1994	CABG	60 (−15)	1) TENS 278 Hz, 60 μs Strong but comfortable 2) Placebo TENS Duration 1 and 2 = 48 hours 3) Control	2 electrodes 2 cm from suture line 2 electrodes either side of T1–T5	TENS vs control – sig lower rest pain in TENS group

Abbreviations:
Inc = increase; **Int** = intensity; **Tol** = tolerable; **Sig** = significant.
Note: the number in brackets in the 'n' column indicates the number of patients who did not complete the study.

difference between groups for pulmonary function (determined by FEV_1 and FVC) nor for opiate requirement. However, the TENS group showed significantly less resting and deep breathing pain scores on the 2nd postoperative day ($p < 0.05$) and less cough pain on the 5th postoperative day ($p < 0.05$) compared to the control group. These results appear somewhat conflicting in that although pain scores were less in the TENS group on certain days, this apparently did not have any overall effect on pulmonary function tests between the two groups.

Postoperative TENS has also been applied for spinal surgical procedures. Issenman et al (1985) gave a retrospective report on a sample of 20 patients who underwent spinal fixation with Harrington rods. Details of pain medication intake on the 4th postoperative day were obtained from the charts of 10 patients who used TENS supplemented by pain medication. Data from a comparison group of 10 age- and sex-matched patients who only received pain medication were also used. Details of TENS parameters were vague; the authors only indicated that pulse duration and frequency parameters were preset and maintained in the mid range for all patients. Comparison of a range of common drugs administered to the patients in both groups showed that the TENS patients used fewer doses than the controls. The authors addressed the limitations of their work in focusing on medication intake on only 1 specific day; this is an example of a study where specific details of parameters are certainly warranted.

Staying in the area of back surgery, a comparatively more detailed study was conducted by McCallum et al (1988) on a group of lumbar laminectomy patients (n = 20). Active TENS (70 Hz, 180 μs) and placebo TENS patients were compared in terms of the number of demands for patient-controlled analgesia during the first 24 postoperative hours. The authors concluded that TENS was no better than a placebo TENS as there were no significant differences between the two groups.

The final study in this section reported the effect of active TENS, placebo TENS and epidural analgesia on pain and ability to contract the quadriceps muscle after knee surgery (Arvidsson & Eriksson 1986). 1 day after surgery, a group of 15 patients performed quadriceps muscle contractions after three different treatments: 15–20 minutes of placebo TENS, 15–20 minutes of active TENS and an epidural injection of local anaesthetic into the knee. All patients received the three treatments in this order. Pain scores were recorded at rest and after muscle contraction; in addition, integrated EMG values recorded during maximum voluntary contraction were used as a measure of contraction ability. Two pairs of electrodes were used for TENS treatment: one pair was applied to the medial and lateral sides of the knee and a second pair applied on the back at the level of L3–L4 (the L3 and L4 dermatomes correspond to the knee region). Pain score results showed that the epidural injection was most effective, giving a 90% reduction in rest pain, active TENS gave a 50% reduction, while placebo TENS actually increased rest pain by 19%. Integrated EMG values showed similar trends; epidural injection produced the largest increase in activity during quadriceps contraction (mean increase of 1846%), TENS produced a mean increase of 305%, while the majority of patients showed a decrease in maximum voluntary contraction after placebo TENS.

The majority of the studies in this section have shown favourable responses to postoperative TENS. Treatment regimes varied considerably in the reviewed studies, e.g. treatment time was either for very short periods of time or continuous throughout the entire postoperative period. In addition, several studies failed to report specific parameter details. In view of the unwanted side-effects accompanying standard narcotic management of postoperative pain, TENS should be considered as a supplement to routine postoperative analgesic management.

Other pain conditions

The sections above have summarised the application of TENS in five common clinical conditions. The efficacy of TENS for pain relief in the following conditions has also been examined:

- myofascial pain syndromes (Graff-Radford et al 1989, Phero et al 1987)
- phantom limb pain (Carabelli & Kellerman 1985, Katz & Melzack 1991)
- orofacial pain (Mehta et al 1994, O'Neil 1981).

SUMMARY OF KEY POINTS

1. Randomised controlled clinical trials are generally regarded as the most effective means of examining treatment efficacy.

2. Many of the studies reviewed in this chapter failed to provide details of treatment parameters and duration of treatment which makes interpretation of results difficult and replication of the study impossible.

3. A large number of the studies in this chapter used acupuncture points as electrode placement sites with considerable success.

4. As many of the reviewed studies produced inconclusive results, this highlights the need for further controlled clinical research on TENS.

REFERENCES

Arvidsson I, Eriksson E 1986 Postoperative TENS pain relief after knee surgery: objective evaluation. Orthopedics 9(10): 1346–1351

Augustinsson L-E, Bohlin P, Bundsen P et al 1977 Pain relief during delivery by chronic low back pain transcutaneous electrical nerve stimulation. Pain 4: 59–65

Bayindir O, Paker T, Akpinar B, Erenturk S, Askin D, Aytac A 1991 Use of transcutaneous electrical nerve stimulation in the control of postoperative chest pain after cardiac surgery. Journal of Cardiothoracic and Vascular Anesthesia 5(6): 589–591

Beard R W, Pearce S 1989 Gynaecological pain. In: Wall P D, Melzack R (eds) Textbook of pain, 2nd edn. Churchill Livingstone, Edinburgh

Bortoluzzi G 1989 Transcutaneous electrical nerve stimulation in labour: practicality and effectiveness in a public hospital ward. Australian Journal of Physiotherapy 35(2): 81–87

Bruce J R, Riggin C S, Parker J C et al 1988 Pain management in rheumatoid arthritis: cognitive behavior modification and transcutaneous neural stimulation. Arthritis Care and Research 1: 78–84

Bundsen P, Ericson K 1982 Pain relief in labour by transcutaneous electrical nerve stimulation – safety aspects. Acta Obstetricia et Gynaecologica Scandinavica 61: 1–5

Bundsen P, Peterson L-E, Selstam U 1981 Pain relief in labor by transcutaneous electrical nerve stimulation. Acta Obstetricia et Gynaecologica Scandinavica 60: 459–468

Bundsen P, Peterson L-E, Selstam U 1982 Pain relief during delivery. Acta Obstetricia et Gynaecologica Scandinavica 61: 289–297

Carabelli R A, Kellerman W C 1985 Phantom limb pain: relief by application of TENS to contralateral extremity. Archives of Physical Medicine and Rehabilitation 66: 466–467

Dawood M Y, Ramos J 1990 Transcutaneous electrical nerve stimulation (TENS) for the treatment of primary dysmenorrhea: a randomised crossover comparison with placebo TENS and ibuprofen. Obstetrics and Gynaecology 75(4): 656–660

Deyo R A, Walsh N E, Martin D C, Schoenfield L S, Ramamurthy S 1990 A controlled trial of transcutaneous electrical nerve stimulation (TENS) and exercise for chronic low back pain. New England Journal of Medicine 322(23): 1627–1634

Ernst E, Resch K L 1996 The clinical trial – gold standard or naive reductionism? European Journal of Physical Medicine and Rehabilitation 6(1): 26–27

Fargas-Babjak A M, Pomeranz B, Rooney P J 1992 Acupuncture-like stimulation with Codetron for rehabilitation of patients with chronic pain syndrome and osteoarthritis. Acupuncture and Electro-Therapeutics Research International Journal 17: 99–105

Forster E L, Kramer J F, Lucy S D, Scudds R A, Novick R J 1994 Effect of TENS on pain, medications and pulmonary function following coronary artery bypass graft surgery. Chest 106(5): 1343–1348

Fox E J, Melzack R 1976 Transcutaneous electrical stimulation and acupuncture: comparison of treatment for low-back pain. Pain 2: 141–148

Graff-Radford S B, Reeves J L, Baker R L, Chiu D 1989 Effects of transcutaneous electrical nerve stimulation on myofascial pain and trigger point sensitivity. Pain 37: 1–5

Grimmer K 1992 A controlled double blind study comparing the effects of strong burst mode TENS and high rate TENS on painful osteoarthritic knees. Australian Journal of Physiotherapy 38(1): 49–56

Harrison R F, Woods T, Shore M, Mathews G, Unwin A 1986 Pain relief in labour using transcutaneous electrical nerve stimulation (TENS): a TENS/TENS placebo controlled study in two parity groups. British Journal of Obstetrics and Gynecology 93: 739–746

Harrison R F, Shore M, Woods T, Mathews G, Gardiner J, Unwin A 1987 A comparative study of transcutaneous electrical nerve stimulation (TENS), entonox, pethidine + promazine and lumbar epidural for pain relief in labor. Acta Obstetricia et Gynaecologica Scandinavica 66: 9–14

Herman E, Williams R, Stratford P, Fargas-Babjak A, Trott M 1994 A randomised controlled trial of transcutaneous electrical nerve stimulation (CODETRON) to determine its benefits in a rehabilitation program for acute occupational low back pain. Spine 19(5): 561–568

Ho A, Hui P W, Cheung J, Cheung C 1987 Effectiveness of transcutaneous electrical nerve stimulation in relieving pain following thoracotomy. Physiotherapy 73(1): 33–35

Issenman J, Nolan M F, Rowley J, Hobby R 1985 Transcutaneous electrical nerve stimulation for pain control after spinal fusion with Harrington rods. Physical Therapy 65(10): 1517–1520

Jensen H, Zesler R, Christensen T 1991 Transcutaneous electrical nerve stimulation (TNS) for painful osteoarthrosis of the knee. International Journal of Rehabilitation Research 14: 356–358

Kaplan B, Peled Y, Pardo J et al 1994 Transcutaneous electrical nerve stimulation (TENS) as a relief for dysmenorrhea. Clinical and Experimental Obstetrics and Gynaecology 21(2): 87–90

Katz J, Melzack R 1991 Auricular transcutaneous electrical nerve stimulation (TENS) reduces phantom limb pain. Journal of Pain and Symptom Management 6(2): 73–83

Laitinen J 1976 Acupuncture and transcutaneous electric stimulation in the treatment of chronic sacrolumbalgia and ischialgia. American Journal of Chinese Medicine 4(2): 169–175

Laitinen J, Nuutinen L 1991 Failure of transcutaneous electrical nerve stimulation and indomethacin to reduce opiate requirement following cholecystectomy. Acta Anaesthesiologica Scandinavica 35: 700–705

Langley G B, Sheppeard H, Johnson M, Wigley R D 1984 The analgesic effects of transcutaneous electrical nerve stimulation and placebo in chronic pain patients. Rheumatology International 4: 119–123

Lehmann T R, Russell D W, Spratt K F et al 1986 Efficacy of electroacupuncture and TENS in the rehabilitation of chronic low back pain patients. Pain 26: 277–290

Lewis B, Lewis D, Cumming G 1994 The comparative analgesic efficacy of transcutaneous electrical nerve stimulation and a non-steroidal anti-inflammatory drug for painful osteoarthritis. British Journal of Rheumatology 33: 455–460

Lewis D, Lewis B, Sturrock R D 1984 Transcutaneous electrical nerve stimulation in osteoarthrosis: a therapeutic alternative? Annals of the Rheumatic Diseases 43: 47–49

McCallum M I D, Glynn C J, Moore R A, Lammer P, Phillips A M 1988 Transcutaneous electrical nerve stimulation in the management of acute postoperative pain. British Journal of Anaesthesia 61: 308–312

Mannheimer C, Carlsson C-A 1979 The analgesic effect of transcutaneous electrical nerve stimulation (TNS) in patients with rheumatoid arthritis: a comparative study of different pulse patterns. Pain 6: 329–334

Mannheimer J S, Whalen E C 1985 The efficacy of transcutaneous electrical nerve stimulation in dysmenorrhea. Clinical Journal of Pain 1: 75–83

Marchand S, Charest J, Li J, Chenard J-R, Lavignolle B, Laurencelle L 1993 Is TENS purely a placebo effect? A controlled study on chronic low back pain. Pain 54: 99–106

Mehta N, Kugel G, Al Shuria A, Sands M, Forgione A 1994 Effect of electronic anesthesia TENS on TMJ and orofacial pain. Journal of Dental Research 73: 358

Melzack R, Jeans M E, Stratford J G, Monks R C 1980 Ice massage and transcutaneous electrical stimulation: comparison of treatment for low back-pain. Pain 9: 209–217

Melzack R, Vetere P, Finch L 1983 Transcutaneous electrical nerve stimulation for low back pain. Physical Therapy 63(4): 489–493

Milsom I, Hedner N, Mannheimer C 1994 A comparative study of the effect of high-intensity transcutaneous electrical nerve stimulation and oral naproxen on intrauterine pressure and menstrual pain in patients with primary dysmenorrhea. American Journal of Obstetrics and Gynecology 170(1): 123–129

Neighbors L E, Clelland J, Jackson J R, Bergman J, Orr J 1987 Transcutaneous electrical nerve stimulation for pain relief in primary dysmenorrhea. Clinical Journal of Pain 3: 17–22

Nesheim B-I 1981 The use of transcutaneous nerve stimulation for pain relief during labor. Acta Obstetricia et Gynaecologica Scandinavica 60: 13–16

O'Neil 1981 Relief of chronic facial pain by transcutaneous electrical nerve stimulation. British Journal of Oral Surgery 19: 112–115

Phero J C, Prithvi Raj P, McDonald J S 1987 Transcutaneous electrical nerve stimulation and myoneural injection therapy for management of chronic myofascial pain. Dental Clinics of North America 31(4): 703–723

Sim D T 1991 Effectiveness of transcutaneous electrical nerve stimulation following cholecystectomy. Physiotherapy 77(10): 715–722

Smith C R, Lewith G T, Machin D 1983 TNS and osteo-arthritic pain. Physiotherapy 69(7): 266–268

Taylor P, Hallett M, Flaherty L 1981 Treatment of osteoarthritis of the knee with transcutaneous electrical nerve stimulation. Pain 11: 233–240

Thomas I L, Tyle V, Webster J, Neilson A 1988 An evaluation of transcutaneous electrical nerve stimulation for pain relief in labour. Australian and New Zealand Journal of Obstetrics and Gynaecology 28: 182–189

Warfield C A, Stein J M, Frank H A 1985 The effect of transcutaneous electrical nerve stimulation on pain after thoracotomy. Annals of Thoracic Surgery 39(5): 462–465

Introduction 103
Contraindications and precautions with TENS 103
Patient preparation for TENS application 105
Selection of TENS parameters 105
Treatment time 106
Electrode placement sites 106
   Painful area 107
   Peripheral nerve 107
   Spinal nerve roots 107
   Acupuncture, motor and trigger points 108
Electrode arrangement 111
Polarity 111
Application of gel/hydrogel pad 111
Attachment of electrodes 112
Home use of TENS 112
The non-responder 113

Pain measurement and assessment 113
   Body charts 114
   Rating scales 114
   Visual analogue scale 114
   McGill Pain Questionnaire 115

**Examples of TENS application for specific pain
   conditions 115**
Labour pain 115
Postoperative pain 117
Phantom limb pain 118

Case histories 119

Summary of key points 123

7

The clinical application of TENS

INTRODUCTION

This chapter provides the reader with a detailed account of how to use TENS in the clinical setting. Preliminary patient screening procedures are outlined prior to performing a TENS treatment, and the subsequent selection criteria involved in choosing electrode placement sites and stimulation parameters are discussed. The evaluation of a patient's response to TENS is an essential element of any treatment programme and therefore a section on pain assessment is included in this chapter. An overview of the application of TENS for a sample of painful conditions is provided and, finally, the information in this chapter is consolidated by the inclusion of several case histories.

Contraindications and precautions with TENS

As with any electrotherapeutic modality or therapeutic procedure, it is essential to screen potential patients for any contraindications to TENS prior to the initial application. There are only a few contraindications to TENS and common sense prevails with the majority of them. They are as follows:

1. Lack of normal skin sensation over the affected area. A simple sharp/blunt test will determine whether cutaneous innervation to the area is intact. If sensation is absent in a specific area, this does not preclude the patient from treatment with TENS. The electrodes may be

placed proximal, in an area which has intact sensation. The danger of placing electrodes over skin which has a deficient sensation is that greater stimulus intensities will have to be employed, which may cause skin irritation and even a burn. In addition, treatment will be ineffective if the appropriate afferent nerves are not stimulated.

2. Patients who are incompetent or who do not comprehend the therapist's instructions (for example, some children or elderly individuals) should not be treated. If patients are required to operate TENS units themselves, it is desirable that they should be responsible individuals.

3. Electrodes should never be placed on the anterior aspect of the neck over the carotid sinuses because stimulation in this area may cause a drop in blood pressure. (The carotid sinuses are spindle-shaped swellings located at the origin of the internal carotid arteries; they contain baroreceptors which detect changes in blood pressure.) Electrodes should also not be placed over the eyes, which common sense would indicate.

4. Many texts list pregnancy as a contraindication to TENS but this requires clarification. This generally refers to placement of electrodes over the pregnant uterus; however, some sources recommend not using TENS for any painful area during pregnancy despite the fact that no adverse reaction to TENS during pregnancy has been reported to date. Mannheimer & Lampe (1984) have reported the successful use of TENS for low back pain in pregnant women, with no adverse effects or complications. (The use of TENS as a method of analgesia during labour is discussed towards the end of this chapter and clinical studies on obstetric TENS are reviewed in Ch. 6.)

5. Patients with pacemakers are also usually listed as a contraindication to TENS; however, this also requires clarification. A study by Rasmussen et al (1988) tested the effect of TENS in 51 patients who had permanent cardiac pacemakers. A range of electrode placement sites was used and no adverse effects were found in any of the 20 models of pacemaker involved in the study. An earlier report by Eriksson et al (1978) indicated that TENS can interfere with cardiac pacemakers of the synchronous type, but that it is safe to use TENS with asynchronous fixed-rate type pacemakers. However, the latter type of pacemaker is rarely used today.

Chen et al (1990) reported two case studies where pacemaker function was monitored using electrocardiography (ECG) and a Holter monitor during TENS application (a Holter monitor is a small device worn on a patient's belt which records 24-hour ECG activity). In these studies, TENS was applied to the upper back/lumbar region, right side posterior neck and right shoulder. In both cases, extended Holter monitoring showed episodes of pacemaker inhibition; however, neither patient reported any cardiac symptoms during these episodes. The sensitivity of both pacemakers was then decreased and upon further monitoring, no episodes of pacemaker inhibition were found. Therefore, it would be advisable to perform an initial trial with concomitant ECG/Holter monitoring when a patient with a pacemaker is considered for TENS treatment.

The effect of TENS on cardiac function has been investigated further by Buonocore et al (1992). Their study examined the effects of high frequency TENS (110 Hz, 0.1 ms, 30 mins), applied over the left forearm, on heart rate variability and vasal sympathetic outflow in 10 healthy subjects. Results indicated that TENS was not able to induce any kind of modification on the autonomic control of the heart. There was, however, a decrease in the amplitude of the plethysmographic wave recorded from the left third fingertip, indicating an increase in sympathetic outflow in the limb. (The effects of TENS on the sympathetic nervous system are discussed further in Ch. 8.)

6. If the patient has an allergic reaction to the electrode gel or tape, this can usually be ascertained in the first treatment; however, most patients have a good idea of what their own allergies are. A few cases of contact dermatitis from TENS have been reported. Zugerman (1982) reported a case of contact dermatitis in a patient who used rubber electrodes and gel; the author believed that the patient developed dermatitis due to propylene glycol, a common ingredient in TENS gel. Patch tests on the patient's skin with

the gel minus propylene glycol were negative whereas patch tests with the gel (complete) and with propylene glycol on its own were both positive. In cases such as these, Zugerman recommended the use of karaya pads placed between the electrode and the skin. A more recent paper by Dwyer et al (1994) also concluded that propylene glycol was a possible cause of contact dermatitis in a patient who had used gel and carbon rubber electrodes.

Marren et al (1991) reported a case of sensitivity to the hydrogel pads commonly used with carbon rubber electrodes (see Ch. 4, Fig. 4.16). The patient in question developed a reaction 9 months after commencing TENS for lower back pain. Patch testing subsequently showed sensitivity to methacrylate, a substance in the hydrogel pad.

7. Patients who have epilepsy should be treated at the discretion of their clinician. If an epileptic patient were using TENS at home, then the safety aspects of what would happen if they took an epileptic fit during TENS application should be considered.

8. Patients should be advised not to wear TENS while driving or operating machinery.

Patient preparation for TENS application

With these contraindications and precautions in mind, it is up to the therapist concerned to take the patient's assessment details and relevant medical history into consideration before proceeding. If the patient is taking pain medication, the initial TENS trial should be performed when the analgesic effects of the medication have worn off, otherwise a normal analgesic effect of the patient's medication may be mistaken for a positive treatment response. If these details are satisfactory, the TENS treatment should then be adequately explained to the patient; this includes attaching the electrodes over a visible body area (e.g. the arm/forearm) and applying the current to allow the patient to experience the sensation. Quite often, patients will appear relieved when they experience this test stimulus due to fear of the unknown. The patient should be positioned

comfortably with the limb/body part suitably supported. The patient should also be instructed not to move, nor touch the electrodes during the treatment. The skin should be cleansed with an alcohol swab to remove surface lipids. There are several chemical fluids available which the manufacturers advise should be sprayed, or applied to enhance electrode conductivity. However, as with the tape and gel, caution must be taken to ensure these chemical fluids do not cause a skin reaction (see Ch. 4 for further details on causes of skin irritation).

Selection of TENS parameters

Once it has been ascertained from clinical assessment of a patient that TENS treatment is appropriate, the therapist is then faced with the dilemma of selecting a suitable treatment regime. Chapter 3 has detailed the different modes of TENS available. When the therapist is faced with a wide range of stimulation parameters and type of output (e.g. modulated or burst), a number of points must be considered before making a decision:

1. Has the patient responded to TENS before? If so, what were the parameters used? There is no point in re-inventing the wheel and if a patient responds favourably to a set of parameters the treatment should commence with the same set.

2. What type of pain is involved? Both acute and chronic pain can be treated with TENS but quite often the patient's symptoms will dictate which pulse frequency to use. For example, if a patient has sustained an acute soft tissue injury of the shoulder, he may not respond favourably to a low frequency current which would cause pulsing contractions in the already traumatised muscle.

3. With any patient who has not used TENS before, it is advisable to commence treatment using conventional TENS. Most patients find the 'tingling, buzzing' sensation associated with this type of TENS more comfortable than the sensation and muscle contractions experienced with acupuncture-like TENS. If pain relief is achieved with conventional TENS, acupuncture-like TENS

should also be tried for at least one treatment and any variation in the length and amount of analgesia noted. It is a good habit to try out both conventional and acupuncture-like TENS because, quite often, dramatic differences are noted in the same patient.

The intensity of the TENS should be increased slowly and the patient asked to report the onset of any sensation under the electrodes. Once this is reported, ask the patient to describe what he feels – it is a useful tip to use the patient's own descriptor when explaining that the intensity will be increased slowly until this sensation is 'strong but comfortable'. Typically, patients will use the words 'tingling, buzzing, pricking, vibration or tapping' to describe the sensation experienced. The patient should be warned that if the intensity is too high then the most beneficial effects will not be achieved. In the application of acupuncture-like TENS the production of muscle contractions is desirable but the patient should be able to tolerate the intensity.

Treatment time

The first TENS trial should be kept short – less than 30 minutes. This treatment time will allow the patient to get used to the sensation but also allows the therapist to monitor any adverse reactions, such as allergies to electrode tape/gel, or if the patient simply cannot tolerate electrical stimulation. After the initial trial, the TENS treatment can be increased to 1 hour at a time at subsequent visits to the therapist. Personal experience has lead the author to advise a maximum treatment period of 1 hour at a time; if TENS is being used at home, the patient should be advised to use the TENS as often as required but only for 1 hour at a time. If a unit is worn for several consecutive hours, as some texts recommend, the skin underneath the electrodes often gets irritated, but even taking half-hour breaks between applications reduces the likelihood of skin irritation. With acupuncture-like TENS, remember that the patient will experience muscle contractions and therefore, with prolonged stimulation, they may experience muscle fatigue –

another good reason for advising a maximum treatment time of only approximately 1 hour at a time.

It is very important that the clinician explains to the patient why TENS should not be continuous. Often patients are tempted to resume otherwise painful functional activities while wearing TENS, and these exacerbate the underlying cause of the pain (e.g. attempting to paint a ceiling while recovering from an acute whiplash!). However, there are two good examples of conditions where TENS is applied continuously: labour pain and postoperative pain. Both are examples of acute pain and are of relatively short duration. (The clinical studies conducted in this area are discussed in more detail in Ch. 6.)

Electrode placement sites

One of the primary factors responsible for a poor response to TENS treatment is that of ineffective electrode placement. No conclusive evidence has emerged from the surprisingly few studies (clinical or experimental) that have investigated the effect of electrode placement on the outcome of TENS treatment (Wheeler et al 1984; Wolf et al 1981). The therapist must be prepared to try several sites before deciding on an optimal placement site, and thus some degree of 'trial and error' is involved in this aspect of the treatment regime. The optimal electrode site not only varies between the conditions to be treated but will also vary between individual patients. Consequently, it should be explained to patients that a few treatments are required initially to locate an effective electrode site for their symptoms and that this period of 'trial and error' will ultimately serve to provide a more successful treatment.

Essentially, there are four broad categories of anatomical site to which TENS electrodes can be applied: painful area, peripheral nerve, spinal nerve roots and other specific points (acupuncture, trigger and motor points). Irrespective of the electrode site that is chosen, stimulation will ultimately result in the passage of afferent information into the central nervous system. In each of the four categories, an appropriate degree of anatomical knowledge is essential in order to achieve effective stimulation.

Painful area

The most commonly used electrode site, which is almost invariably the first choice of most clinicians, is that over or close to the painful area itself. In particular, since it is desirable with conventional TENS to achieve a sensation of paraesthesia over the affected area, this may involve placement of electrodes at proximal and distal ends of the painful area. As previously outlined, skin sensation must be assessed before TENS can be applied in order to ensure normal innervation of the affected area. This may apparently pose a potential problem in those patients in whom sensation is diminished or absent in the affected area. However, in such cases, the electrodes can be placed just proximal to this site (over normal innervated skin) in order to stimulate the afferent sensory nerves travelling to the spinal cord from the affected area; thus effective treatment can be given even where there is diminished sensation. There are also occasions when application of electrodes at the painful site would prove to be uncomfortable to the patient, as in the case of hypersensitivity following a peripheral nerve injury. In such situations, it may also be more appropriate to place the electrodes proximal to the area of hypersensitivity.

Peripheral nerve

The electrodes may also be placed over a peripheral nerve which has a cutaneous distribution in the painful area. Peripheral nerves (e.g. median and sciatic nerves) arise from plexuses in the cervical, lumbar and sacral regions of the spinal cord; there are no such plexuses in the thoracic region. These plexuses are formed by the union of the ventral rami of spinal nerves. A sound knowledge of surface marking and neuroanatomy is required to determine where the peripheral nerves are most superficial and therefore most easily accessible for stimulation. For example, pain experienced on the dorsum of the lateral aspect of the hand and the first and second

digits can be treated with electrodes placed over the superficial radial nerve which runs along the lateral aspect of the lower one-third of the forearm. Other examples of superficial points of peripheral nerves are the ulnar groove for the ulnar nerve and the head of the fibula for the common peroneal nerve. The electrodes should be placed directly over the appropriate nerve where it runs a more superficial course.

Spinal nerve roots

31 pairs of spinal nerves emerge from the vertebral column via the intervertebral foramina. Each spinal nerve is formed by the union of ventral (motor) and dorsal (sensory) roots which unite in the intervertebral foramen to form a mixed spinal nerve. The intervertebral foramina lie between the non-palpable transverse processes of the vertebral column (Fig. 7.1). By placing the electrodes parallel to the vertebral column (paraspinal application) and over the intervertebral foramina, this will allow for stimulation of the appropriate roots of spinal nerves which supply the affected dermatome (i.e. the area of skin which receives its nerve supply from a specified spinal nerve) or myotome (i.e. groups of muscles supplied by a specified spinal nerve). Acupuncture-like TENS is commonly applied to myotomes segmentally related to the area of pain to produce the desirable muscle contractions associated with this mode of TENS. There is considerable overlap between adjacent dermatomes in a specified body part (Fig. 7.2) and knowledge of the spinal nerve responsible for the dermatome in question is required in order accurately to select the correct spinal segment for stimulation.

A knowledge of the relationship between spinal cord segments, their corresponding spinal nerves and the spinal vertebral processes is also important. For example, in the cervical column there are eight cervical spinal nerves and only seven cervical vertebrae so the seventh cervical nerve will emerge between the seventh cervical and first thoracic vertebrae. It is important to remember that due to the different posterior angulation of the vertebral spinous processes in

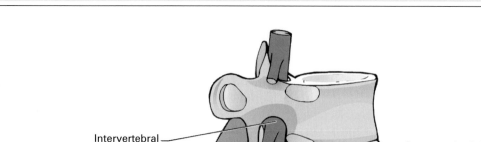

Figure 7.1 Lateral view of two thoracic vertebrae illustrating a spinal nerve emerging via the intervertebral foramen.

each section of the vertebral column (see Fig. 7.3), palpation of a specific spinous process does not necessarily mean that placement of an electrode just lateral to the process will stimulate the nerve roots of that particular spinal nerve (e.g., in the cervical spine, palpation of C5 spinous process corresponds to the level at which the C6 nerve root emerges).

The problem of accurate electrode placement is overcome to a degree by the fact that the length of standard electrodes (~5 cm) allows at least two adjacent roots to be stimulated simultaneously, although it should be stressed that this fact does not obviate the need for accurate palpation and care in placement of electrodes. It is also important to place the electrodes parallel to the spinal column and not in a transverse direction, in order to ensure stimulation of a maximum number of nerve roots (Fig. 7.4).

Acupuncture, motor and trigger points

The final category of site for electrode placement is a group of points referred to as *specific points*, of which there are essentially three types – acupuncture, motor and trigger points. A motor point is the point of entry of a motor nerve into a muscle and is characterised by high electrical conductance and low skin resistance. Motor points are thus used for optimal stimulation of a muscle and therefore may be effectively employed as electrode placement sites when applying acupuncture-like TENS, when muscle contraction is desirable (see Ch. 3).

Trigger points and acupuncture points are also frequently used as sites for electrostimulation in experimental and clinical studies as well as routine clinical practice. Trigger points are areas characterised by tenderness on palpation and the production of referred pain; they are found in skeletal muscles, tendons, joint capsules, ligaments, the periosteum and the skin (Baldry 1989). In contrast, acupuncture points are well defined specific points along so-called meridians on the body which traditional Chinese medicine (TCM) asserts can be stimulated to treat disease; disease in this case is proposed to be due to the imbalance of 'yin' and 'yang', and stimulation of certain points can improve the flow of 'chi energy' and thus treat the disease.

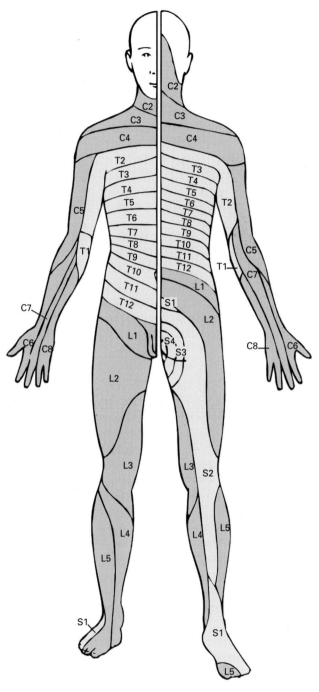

Figure 7.2 Dermatomes on the anterior and posterior aspect of the body.

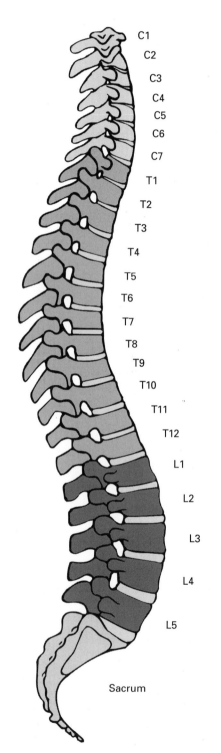

Figure 7.3 Lateral view of the spinal column illustrating the angulation of the spinous processes in each region.

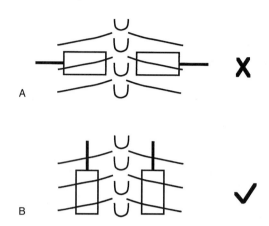

Figure 7.4 Application of electrodes parallel to the spinal column ensures stimulation of a maximum number of spinal nerves.

While a more comprehensive account of acupuncture as a general treatment is beyond the scope of this text, this is well covered elsewhere (see, for example, Baldry 1989). Fine metal needles are usually employed to stimulate such points; however, a variety of other techniques (electrical, laser, pressure) have been used to stimulate both trigger and acupuncture points for pain relief (Haker & Lundeberg 1990, Laitinen 1976). Many clinicians advocate the use of these points as they are easy to locate by palpation and subjective report of local tenderness. Melzack et al (1977) compared the spatial distribution and associated pain patterns of trigger points and traditional acupuncture points, using body maps compiled by several authors, and concluded that there was a high degree of correspondence (71%) for both criteria. Several clinical studies have reported the success of TENS application over these specific points (Fox & Melzack 1976, Laitinen 1976), all of which have some degree of decreased resistance to electrical currents, and thus represent ideal sites for electrical stimulation.

The ultimate choice of electrode site depends upon accurate assessment of the cause and location of the pain and also the type of TENS to be used. If conventional TENS is used, the desired sensation is that of a comfortable paraesthesia; it follows, therefore, that it is undesirable to place the electrodes over a bony prominence (e.g. the malleoli), as this would produce a rather un-comfortable sensation for the patient. In contrast, when acupuncture-like TENS is used, it is desirable to produce visible muscle contractions (as outlined in Ch. 3), and therefore placement of electrodes should be over a muscle related to the area of pain (the appropriate motor point/myotome can be used).

Electrode arrangement

Electrodes may be placed unilaterally or bilaterally, depending on the site of the pain and its origin: for example, treatment of low back pain due to degenerative changes of the lumbar spine would involve bilateral paraspinal application of electrodes at the appropriate segmental level (i.e. parallel to the vertebral column), whereas unilateral application would be more appropriate for pain in the right shoulder related to a soft tissue injury. Many TENS units have dual or indeed multiple channels which may be used effectively for pain of multiple origin/location. If it has been ascertained that there is referred pain resulting from irritation of a specific nerve, for example the sciatic nerve, then a dual channel unit may be utilised to place one channel paraspinally at the level of origin of the sciatic nerve (L4, L5, S1, S2 and S3) and a second channel at the site of referred pain (e.g. posterior thigh).

Other possible electrode arrangements include the following:

• A two-channel criss-cross arrangement. This arrangement would be appropriate for diffuse joint pain as all aspects of the joint are being treated. This type of electrode arrangement has also been used successfully for the management of dysmenorrhoea by placing the electrodes over the abdomen (see Ch. 6 for details).

• Application of the electrodes on the contralateral limb. In cases of phantom limb pain, the stump is often too sensitive for ipsilateral electrode placement: the electrodes can be placed either over the appropriate spinal nerve roots or other peripheral sites on the contralateral limb so that the incoming neural traffic resulting from stimulation arrives at the spinal segment which supplies the amputated limb.

Polarity

With regard to electrode polarity (discussed in Ch. 3), there is relatively little literature available advocating preferential placement of anode or cathode. However, since the cathode is the active electrode, in stimulation of a nerve fibre it follows that it should always be placed proximal (i.e. closest to the spinal cord) in order to prevent *anodal block*. As described in Chapter 3, depolarisation takes place under the cathode whereas hyperpolarisation occurs under the anode. This hyperpolarisation displaces the nerve membrane potential further away from the threshold for activation and may impede the conduction of an action potential, hence the term 'anodal block' (Swett & Bourassa 1981). Essentially, this means that a greater amount of current (intensity of stimulation) is required to stimulate a nerve under the anode than one under the cathode. Because of this effect, where possible, the cathode should be applied nearest (i.e. proximal to the anode) the desired destination of the action potential (i.e. the spinal cord). The cathode should also be placed directly over the motor point or specific point if this is chosen as the appropriate stimulation site, since less current is required for stimulation. Indeed, patients commonly report stronger sensation under one electrode than under the other – this stronger sensation is usually felt under the cathode.

Application of gel/hydrogel pad

If wet gel is used, care must be taken to spread it evenly over the surface of the electrode (this is most easily done with a clean finger). Alternatively, if a hydrogel pad is used, ensure that there are no air bubbles. The hydrogel pads are usually packaged between two sheets of plastic (see Fig. 4.16). The easiest way to apply a pad to a carbon rubber electrode is to peel off one of the sheets of plastic and then place the electrode on top of the exposed hydrogel pad. Any air bubbles should be removed before discarding the second plastic sheet, by applying pressure with a thumb towards the periphery of the electrode.

Attachment of electrodes

Chapter 4 illustrated some of the variety of TENS electrodes that are currently available. If micropore tape is used to secure electrodes, as in a carbon rubber electrode and gel application, it is important that the strips of tape cover the electrode evenly (as indicated in Fig. 7.5), which ensures uniform skin–electrode contact. One central strip of tape should not be used because this causes uneven skin–electrode contact and thus affects current distribution. The tape should be removed in the direction of the hair growth in the area, both to avoid discomfort to the patient and also to reduce the possibility of skin irritation/infection due to the removal of body hair. In some cases it may be appropriate to shave body hair before applying the electrodes if it prevents tape or electrodes from adhering. It is important to know that interelectrode distance will affect both the current density and depth of penetration of the current. Current density (the amount of current per unit area) decreases with

distance from the electrodes due to a high electrical impedance of the deeper tissues. If the interelectrode distance is decreased, current density in the area between the electrodes will increase and the depth of penetration will decrease. Conversely, with a greater interelectrode distance the current density is less but the depth of penetration is greater. As a guideline, the interelectrode distance should ideally be at least equal to the diameter of the electrode, in order to avoid excessive current density between the electrodes (Mannheimer & Lampe 1984).

With the above factors in mind, it is advisable to commence a course of treatment with electrode placement over the painful area, as this usually results in the production of hypoalgesia in the affected painful area. Then, depending on the results of this application, the therapist may choose alternative sites from the selection of electrode placement sites described earlier (e.g. peripheral nerve, special points). It is imperative to take the patient's comfort into account when selecting the treatment regime. For example, electrode placement around the shoulder girdle usually gives rise to a certain degree of muscle activity due to the density of motor points in the area. (This typically occurs with a low pulse frequency but can also occur with a high frequency if high current intensities are used.) Many patients find this muscle activity unpleasant and so placement of electrodes over the spinal nerve roots at the corresponding segmental level would be a more satisfactory treatment arrangement for these patients. Feedback from the patient is an essential element in the selection of an optimal electrode placement site.

Home use of TENS

If the therapist recommends home use of TENS, a relative or carer should be present when instruction is given. The patient should be given a few electrode placement sites to try. It should be stressed that the TENS unit is for the patient's use only and that nobody else, friend or relative, should be given the TENS unit to 'try out' if they have not been properly assessed or advised by a qualified clinician. Before going home with the

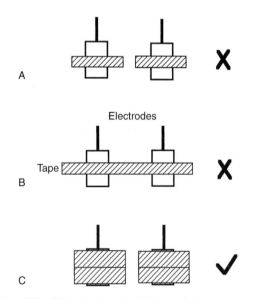

Figure 7.5 Adhesive tape should be applied evenly across the TENS electrodes and not just across the centre which would result in unequal distribution of current.

unit, the patient should experience the sensation in whatever position he will be applying it at home; if he intends wearing it around the house he will benefit from experiencing how the current intensity can alter on transferring positions, etc. If this is demonstrated adequately, it will save a considerable amount of the therapist's and patient's time dealing with subsequent queries of concern from the patient.

Floter (1986) highlighted the fact that a high percentage of patients who are non-responders to home use of TENS simply do not use the unit. In his study of 151 patients, he monitored home use of TENS by a timing device in the TENS unit which recorded hours of operation. Out of 65 patients who failed to obtain adequate pain relief, only 10 had used the TENS on a regular basis. This observation really highlights the fact that clinicians need to be assured of their patients' motivation before issuing a TENS for home use. Some of the units described in Chapter 10 have a 'use meter' which allows the clinician to monitor the time the unit is used by the patient at home.

The contraindications and precautions outlined in an earlier section of this chapter specifically emphasise that patients should not use a TENS unit when driving or operating machinery. It is quite possible for a patient receiving TENS to the lumbar spine to experience a sudden increase in current intensity due to sudden braking while driving; it follows that wearing TENS while driving is a potential hazard. This sudden increase in current intensity can be easily demonstrated by asking the patient to sit in a forward lean position and then extend his trunk so that his back makes contact with the back of the chair.

The non-responder

A certain percentage of patients who have TENS treatment will not respond positively. This must be borne in mind if a therapist has exhausted all possible combinations of stimulation parameters and electrode sites with no beneficial effects. TENS should not be given as an isolated treatment. A series of appropriate exercises, postural advice and other therapeutic procedures may be included in the patient's overall treatment programme.

A recent study by Marchand et al (1995) has indicated that caffeine may reduce the analgesic effects of TENS. They investigated the effect of 200 mg of placebo and 200 mg caffeine on the analgesic effect of TENS, using thermally-induced pain in healthy subjects. After caffeine, TENS had no effect on the intensity and unpleasantness of thermal pain; however, after placebo both were significantly reduced. The authors concluded that TENS analgesia may be mediated by adenosine because caffeine is an adenosine-receptor antagonist; furthermore, they suggested that TENS analgesia may be enhanced by a reduction in caffeine intake. This relationship between caffeine and TENS analgesia may be responsible for a certain percentage of non-responders and certainly warrants further investigation.

PAIN MEASUREMENT AND ASSESSMENT

In any course of treatment, objective and subjective data are required to monitor a patient's response to the treatment. In the case of pain measurement, methods of assessment range in complexity from simply asking a patient to rate their current pain 'out of 10' to a detailed questionnaire and body chart type of assessment. The choice is really up to the individual clinician. There are, however, a number of guidelines which may assist in selecting an appropriate assessment to measure a response to TENS treatment. First:

● Make sure the method of measurement is standardised so that if a different clinician takes over the treatment, they may continue the procedure without difficulty.

● If measurement is required for a clinical trial or experimental pain study, it is imperative that data can be obtained which can be easily analysed for the purposes of statistical analysis.

The following section briefly describes the more common methods of pain assessment which can be used to evaluate a TENS treatment.

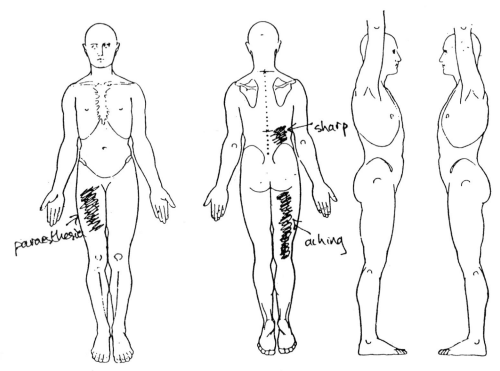

Figure 7.6 A body chart represents a basic method of pain measurement.

Body charts

The distribution of pain can be depicted on a body chart by the patient or clinician (Fig. 7.6). This method of assessment is particularly useful if the patient has a number of painful areas and can be very helpful to demonstrate the progress of a course of treatment from the initial assessment.

Rating scales

Rating scales are common methods of assessing pain because they are simple, economical and easy to understand (Chapman et al 1985). The patient can be asked to choose from a range of descriptive words (verbal rating scale) or from a scale of 1 to 10/100 (numerical rating scale) to describe their pain intensity.

Visual analogue scale

The most simple and indeed reliable form of pain measurement is the visual analogue scale (VAS, see Fig. 7.7). It consists of a 10 cm line which has the words 'no pain' or 'I do not have any pain' marked at one extremity and 'pain at its worst' or 'my pain could not be worse' marked at the other extremity (Echternach 1987). The patient is asked to mark the 10 cm line at the point which represents their 'current pain' intensity. The distance between the 'no pain' end to the patient's mark is measured and this provides a pain intensity score. There is considerable evidence to suggest that the VAS fulfils the majority of the criteria for an ideal method of pain measurement (Price 1985). Wallenstein (1984) found a consistent relationship between VAS and verbal scales which serves to heighten the validity and reliability of both measures. The overall ad-

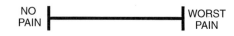

NO PAIN |————————————————| WORST PAIN

Figure 7.7 A visual analogue scale.

vantages of the VAS compared to other rating scales are its simplicity, sensitivity and speed of completion.

McGill Pain Questionnaire

Rating scales have the limitation that they tend to only quantify pain intensity, whereas the McGill Pain Questionnaire (MPQ) quantifies the sensory, affective and evaluative dimensions of the pain experience; hence this popular method of pain measurement is recognised as a multidimensional pain questionnaire (Chen & Treede 1985, DiGregorio et al 1991). 20 groups of words are presented in the questionnaire (Fig. 7.8), each group describing a different dimension of pain. There are four classes of pain descriptors incorporated in the questionnaire (Melzack 1975):

1. Sensory – words that relate the temporal, spatial, thermal and other sensory qualities of pain.
2. Affective – words that describe tension, fear and autonomic qualities of pain are included in this class.
3. Evaluative – words that describe the subjective intensity of the pain.
4. Miscellaneous – this class contains those words that don't belong in any of the other three classes.

The questionnaire is administered as follows: the patient chooses one word from each group which most accurately describes the pain they experienced; if no word is appropriate in a particular group, then no word is ticked. The words within each group are assigned rank orders, therefore a score can be obtained from the words chosen. Four main measures of pain may be obtained from the questionnaire (Melzack 1975):

1. Pain rating index (PRI) – this is the sum of the rank values assigned to each word which depends upon its position in each sub-group. Scores can be obtained for each of the four classes of pain as outlined above as well as an overall total score (PRI).
2. A second PRI score which is the sum total of scale values in one particular group or for all

the groups (based on the earlier work of Melzack & Torgerson 1971).

3. Present pain intensity (PPI) – this measures overall pain intensity on a scale of 0–5 at the time of administration of the questionnaire.

4. Number of words chosen (NWC).

EXAMPLES OF TENS APPLICATION FOR SPECIFIC PAIN CONDITIONS

This section discusses the application of TENS for three different types of pain. (See Ch. 6 for an in-depth review of a range of clinical studies that have been conducted on TENS.)

Labour pain

In the survey of chartered physiotherapists discussed in Chapter 1, 85.5% of respondents ranked TENS first against six other electrotherapeutic modalities for obstetric pain. The intensity of labour pain has been ranked higher than several clinical pain syndromes including arthritis, postherpetic neuralgia and phantom limb pain (Melzack et al 1981). The primary factor to be considered with selection of any type of analgesia during labour is the potential side-effects of the intervention on both the foetus and the mother. Entonox (50:50 mixture of nitrous oxide and oxygen), intramuscular or intravenous narcotics and epidural blocks are examples of standard methods of obstetric analgesia. TENS has several advantages over other types of obstetric analgesia in that it is non-invasive, it gives the mother a level of control and she remains fully alert during the birth. Furthermore, the safety of TENS has also been investigated and no adverse effects observed in either mother or foetus in several studies (Bundsen & Ericson 1982, Harrison et al 1986).

An obstetric TENS is usually introduced to the mother-to-be in the antenatal class by the physiotherapist or midwife. Prospective mothers are given a demonstration of TENS and if they wish to use it they will usually take a unit home to practice using it with their partner. Figure 7.9 illustrates the areas and intensity of pain typically experienced during the stages of labour.

McGill Pain Questionnaire

Patient's Name _____ Date _____ Time_____am/pm

PRI: S_____ A_____ E_____ M_____ PRI(T) _____ PPI____
   (1-10)   (11-15)   (16)   (17-20)   (1-20)

1 FLICKERING QUIVERING PULSING THROBBING BEATING POUNDING	11 TIRING EXHAUSTING
2 JUMPING FLASHING SHOOTING	12 SICKENING SUFFOCATING
3 PRICKING BORING DRILLING STABBING LANCINATING	13 FEARFUL FRIGHTFUL TERRIFYING
4 SHARP CUTTING LACERATING	14 PUNISHING GRUELLING CRUEL VICIOUS KILLING
5 PINCHING PRESSING GNAWING CRAMPING CRUSHING	15 WRETCHED BLINDING
6 TUGGING PULLING WRENCHING	16 ANNOYING TROUBLESOME MISERABLE INTENSE UNBEARABLE
7 HOT BURNING SCALDING SEARING	17 SPREADING RADIATING PENETRATING PIERCING
8 TINGLING ITCHY SMARTING STINGING	18 TIGHT NUMB DRAWING SQUEEZING TEARING
9 DULL SORE HURTING ACHING HEAVY	19 COOL COLD FREEZING
10 TENDER TAUT RASPING SPLITTING	20 NAGGING NAUSEATING AGONIZING DREADFUL TORTURING

BRIEF MOMENTARY TRANSIENT | RHYTHMIC PERIODIC INTERMITTENT | CONTINUOUS STEADY CONSTANT

E = EXTERNAL
I = INTERNAL

PPI
0 NO PAIN
1 MILD
2 DISCOMFORTING
3 DISTRESSING
4 HORRIBLE
5 EXCRUCIATING

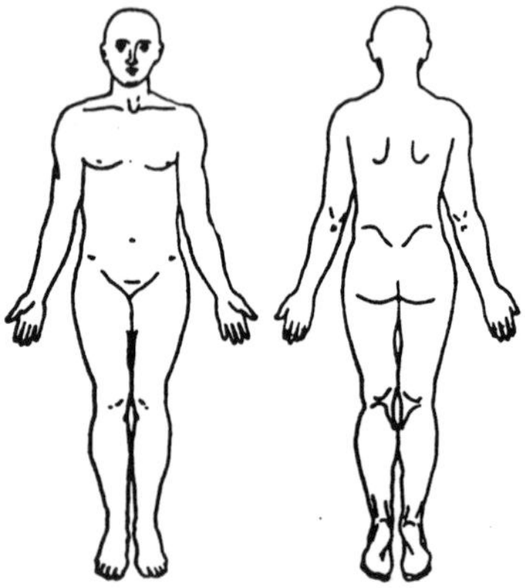

COMMENTS:

Figure 7.8 The McGill Pain Questionnaire. (Reproduced from Reading 1989; in: Wall & Melzack 1989, with permission.)

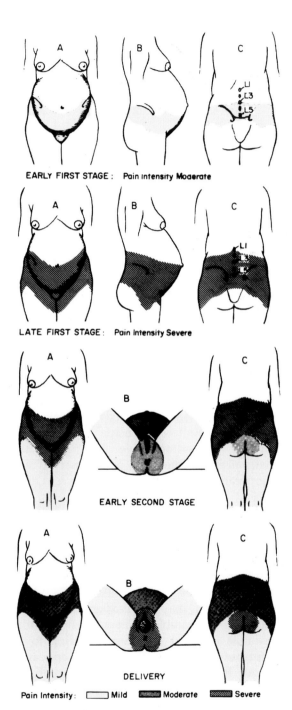

EARLY FIRST STAGE : Pain Intensity Moderate

LATE FIRST STAGE : Pain Intensity Severe

EARLY SECOND STAGE

DELIVERY

Pain Intensity : ☐ Mild ▨ Moderate ▩ Severe

Figure 7.9 The intensity and distribution of labour pain during the various phases of labour and delivery. (Reproduced from Bonica & Chadwick 1989; in: Wall & Melzack 1989, with permission.)

Standard electrode placement sites are used for labour pain. Two pairs of electrodes are placed over the spinal nerve roots at the level of T10–L1 and S2–S4 (see Fig. 7.10), therefore a dual channel unit is required; the lower electrodes are usually slightly shorter in length. These two spinal levels are used because they receive incoming nociceptive information from the uterus, cervix and perineal structures.

A typical obstetric TENS has both continuous and burst outputs; the continuous output is used during contractions and the burst output is used between contractions. The frequency can be variable or fixed; if it is fixed it is usually set at approximately 80–100 Hz and the burst output typically has a frequency of two bursts per second.

Most obstetric TENS units have a 'boost' control which allows the user to switch between the continuous and burst outputs (in earlier units the switch changed the intensity level). This is shaped so that the patient can easily hold it in her hand with a button at the top which is pressed to switch the type of output (see Fig. 7.11). A more recent design of obstetric TENS unit (Lifetime Obstetric TENS®, NEEN Healthcare, UK) has incorporated a trigger switch into the base unit instead of the larger boost control (see Ch. 10, Fig. 10.9).

Postoperative pain

Postoperative pain is a good example of an application of TENS for acute pain. The majority of general hospitals routinely use patient-controlled analgesia (PCA) as a method of controlling postoperative pain. This method allows the patient to administer a standardised amount of an analgesic, typically morphine, whenever their pain dictates. The advantages of this system are that it cuts down on staff time and that the patient is very much in control of their pain management. Similarly, postoperative TENS offers the patient a major role in their pain management. Once the patient has been instructed on the operation of the TENS unit and a suitable treatment programme, they are then in charge of this aspect of their postoperative care.

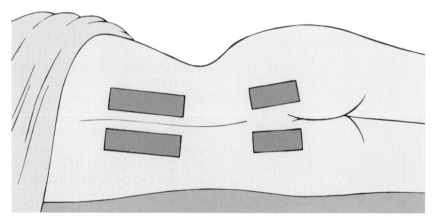

Figure 7.10 Electrode placement sites for labour pain; one pair of electrodes is placed at T10–L1 level and a second pair is placed at the level of S2–S4.

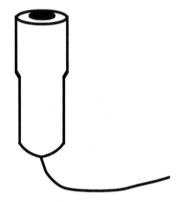

Figure 7.11 A typical 'boost' control which is attached to an obstetric TENS unit.

Several clinical trials have investigated the efficacy of postoperative TENS after a range of surgical procedures including hand surgery, coronary artery bypass graft (CABG) surgery and thoracotomy (Arvidsson & Eriksson 1986, Bourke et al 1984, Forster et al 1994, McMichan et al 1985). Sterile, disposable electrodes placed parallel but a few cm away from the incision appear to produce the best results. A second pair of electrodes can also be placed parallel to the vertebral spinous processes over the spinal nerve roots which correspond to the dermatomes in the area of the incision. In addition, a high frequency, long pulse duration current combined with a comfortable intensity without muscle contractions has been reported to produce the greatest

pain relief (Ho et al 1987, Mannheimer & Lampe 1984).

Postoperative TENS is not usually given in isolation but in addition to standard narcotics. Stimulation usually starts immediately upon return to the recovery room and continues for up to 72 hours post surgery. It has been observed that in addition to providing pain relief, TENS can also indirectly improve lung function because the patient finds it easier to take deep breaths and cough when using the TENS. The reduction of postoperative ileus is another beneficial effect which has been observed with postoperative TENS (Mannheimer & Lampe 1984).

Phantom limb pain

Phantom limb pain is one of the consequences of limb amputation which occurs in 80–100% of amputees (Jensen & Rasmussen 1989). The amputee patient may often experience a combination of unbearable pain and non-painful sensations from an area corresponding to the amputated limb. Conventional TENS appears to produce the best results for this type of pain with electrodes commonly applied to the stump. However, if the stump is hypersensitive, a proximal application of electrodes along peripheral nerves, over spinal nerve roots or indeed on the contralateral limb, may be tried.

CASE HISTORIES

The following five case histories provide examples of TENS applications for a variety of pain conditions. Each case history is accompanied by a photograph to illustrate the electrode placement site.

Case history 1

History

Mrs K., a 32-year-old woman, presented with a 2-year history of constant pain in her right shoulder, thoracic spine and rib cage. The patient thought that the onset of the problem was related to a soft tissue injury of her right shoulder, sustained while cutting a hedge with heavy electric clippers. Several investigative tests were performed (blood tests, chest X-ray, bone scan), none of which showed anything abnormal. The patient was clearly distressed at the lack of a definite diagnosis and was showing signs of depression. She was very anxious and lack of sleep contributed to her distressed appearance. Due to the negative investigative findings, this patient began thinking the pain was 'all in her head'; her GP had prescribed antidepressants which she refused.

Assessment findings

Examination of this patient revealed marked tenderness medial to the right scapula and over the upper and middle fibres of both trapezii. Palpation of the facet joints of the upper to mid thoracic spine on the right produced referred pain around the right rib cage.

Treatment

Six treatments were given over a 3-month period; treatment consisted of posture correction, exercises, acupuncture and home TENS. Acupuncture was applied to LI4 bilaterally and over the tender area medial to the right scapula. The patient responded very well to acupuncture, experiencing almost immediate relief and relaxation. TENS was applied by two self-adhesive elec-

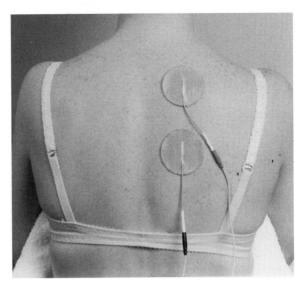

Figure 7.12 Electrode positions for case history 1.

trodes placed over the painful area (medial scapular border; see Fig. 7.12). Stimulation parameters were 200 µs pulse duration, strong but comfortable intensity and variable frequency. Initially, the stimulation frequency was set at 120 Hz, then the patient was advised to switch to low frequency (4 Hz) to compare effects. Mrs K. was told to wear the TENS at home for an hour at a time as often as required.

Treatment outcome

The patient reported that the 'magic box' controlled her pain both at work and at home. Her general appearance markedly improved and she became much more confident about managing her condition. An important factor in the success of her treatment was that she was reassured that she was not imagining her symptoms and that she understood the concept of referred pain. Mrs K. felt that low frequency TENS (approximately 4 Hz) was more comfortable and effective than higher frequencies and therefore she used this frequency setting after an initial trial period. Three months after the first treatment, examination revealed no tenderness over the thoracic spine / related area. The patient had occasional episodes of discomfort in the right shoulder region associated with increased activity but was able to manage this with her TENS which she subsequently purchased.

Case history 2

History

Mr P., a 62-year-old man, fell on his outstretched right (dominant) hand and sustained a Colles fracture along with a fractured scaphoid and ulnar styloid process; he was subsequently immobilised in a below elbow plaster of Paris for 6 weeks. He presented for treatment 3 days after the plaster had been removed.

Assessment findings

Examination of this patient revealed considerable loss of all movements of the wrist joint, supination and thumb opposition. Mr P. was unable to grip and therefore function was severely impaired. His hand was swollen and he reported intermittent rest pain over the ulnar border of the wrist joint and over the scaphoid, which was increased by active movement. Mr P.'s work involved considerable amounts of time using a computer, therefore restoration of full wrist and finger function was imperative.

Treatment

Mr P. was treated over a 6-week period. During the first week, daily treatment was given; this consisted of active exercises, PNF, laser irradiation and TENS. TENS was applied by two self-adhesive electrodes placed proximal and distal to the painful area along the ulnar border (Fig. 7.13). Stimulation parameters were 200 µs pulse duration, 110 Hz frequency and strong but comfortable intensity. After the first week, this patient was treated twice a week. TENS was always applied immediately post exercise/proprioceptive neuromuscular facilitation (PNF) for a 30–40-minute period.

Treatment outcome

This patient was highly motivated to return to

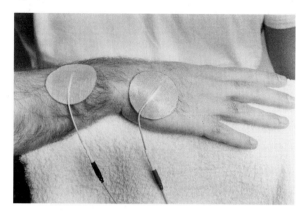

Figure 7.13 Electrode positions for case history 2.

work quickly. Full functional movements were achieved by the third week. The patient's range of movement improved to 95% of full range within the 6 weeks; this was an excellent result considering that there were three fractures in the area. Significant pain relief was obtained with the TENS; at the end of the 6 weeks, the patient reported only a 'mild tightness' over the ulnar border of the wrist on sudden movements of the wrist.

Case history 3

History

Mr S., a 55-year-old man, presented with a 1-week history of sudden onset low back pain sustained when he hyperextended his lumbar spine while fixing a light bulb. This patient had had a history of 'back problems' since he was 16 years old.

Assessment findings

Assessment showed generalised tenderness on palpation of his lumbar spine with no muscle spasm elicited. Active range of lumbar extension was considerably restricted (~50%). There were no neurological signs and there was no referred pain. There was radiological evidence of degenerative changes at L3, L4 and L5 levels. Mr S. reported an aching pain in the centre of his lumbar spine on lifting objects.

Treatment

Treatment consisted of active lumbar extension exercises and TENS. TENS was applied by two carbon rubber electrodes and hydrogel pads positioned bilaterally opposite L3/L4 spinous processes (Fig. 7.14). Stimulation parameters were 200 μs pulse duration, 110 Hz frequency and strong but comfortable intensity. Mr S. received four treatments in total (twice a week for 2 weeks). TENS was applied for 40 minutes on each occasion. Mr S. carried out a home exercise programme of lumbar extension exercises twice a day.

Treatment outcome

The patient's range of lumbar extension returned to full range within the 4 weeks and the lumbar spine pain and tenderness completely resolved.

Case history 4

History

Mrs F., a 44-year-old woman, presented 4 weeks after surgery for carpal tunnel syndrome in her dominant right hand. Mrs F. had been discharged by the surgeon but returned to her GP within 2 weeks complaining of severe functional impairment due to hypersensitivity in the palm of her hand and persistent pain around the scar. By the time she received an appointment, Mrs F. was 5 weeks post surgery.

Assessment findings

Examination of this patient revealed hypersensitivity to touch on the palmar aspect of the hand in the distribution of the median nerve (i.e. lateral two-thirds). The patient could not bear to hold any object in her hand and, as a result of inactivity, her finger flexors had become very weak. There was intermittent aching pain around the scar, just proximal to the wrist; the scar tissue had not been mobilised at any stage post surgery and by the time Mrs F. presented for treatment, it had become quite adherent.

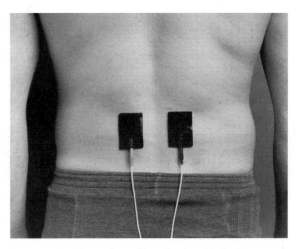

Figure 7.14 Electrode positions for case history 3.

Treatment

Mrs F. was treated twice a week for 6 weeks; treatment consisted of sensory reeducation of the palmar aspect of the hand, functional hand exercises, mobilisation of the scar tissue and TENS. As the area around the scar was not normal upon sharp/blunt testing, the electrodes were applied over the course of the median nerve in the forearm just proximal to the scar. Two carbon rubber electrodes were applied to the skin with gel and micropore tape (see Fig. 7.15 for electrode placement site). The first treatment was limited to only 10 minutes to observe any latent effect of TENS on the hypersensitivity in the hand. After the second treatment of 30 minutes, Mrs F. reported that the sensitivity in her palm felt 'more normal' and that this effect lasted for several hours post treatment. The treatment time was increased to 45 minutes on subsequent days with marked improvements after each treatment. Stimulation parameters were 50 μs pulse duration, 100 Hz frequency and comfortable intensity (i.e. conventional TENS).

Treatment outcome

This patient's functional improvement was associated with a normalisation of sensation in her hand. Conventional TENS produced a comforting normal sensation while it was applied and, over the 6 weeks of treatment, the normal

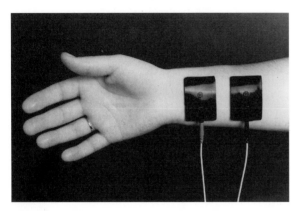

Figure 7.15 Electrode positions for case history 4.

sensation gradually became permanent. In addition, the pain around the scar site also decreased. As the pain decreased, this patient gradually gained strength in her finger flexors.

Case history 5

History

Mrs McC., a 60-year-old woman, presented with typical symptoms of left frozen shoulder of unknown cause. She reported that her left shoulder had become progressively stiff and painful over a 6-week period. Radiographs showed no degenerative changes. She was referred for physiotherapy 6 months after the onset of her symptoms.

Assessment findings

Mrs McC. had 50% restriction of active shoulder flexion, abduction, medial and lateral rotation. There was considerable pain at the end of range of all these movements at the anterior and posterior aspects of the shoulder joint. There was marked tenderness on the anterior aspect of the joint. Mrs McC. had been offered a steroid injection by her GP but refused because she wanted 'to try physiotherapy first'. As she was right-handed she had developed a habit of not trying to use the left hand functionally. Getting dressed was a particular problem for Mrs McC.; in addition, she knitted sweaters as a hobby and was quite depressed that she was unable to pursue this hobby due to pain. This patient could not

sleep at night because she inadvertently rolled onto the left shoulder several times during the night and was woken by the pain.

Treatment

Mrs McC. was treated twice a week for 8 weeks; treatment consisted of active exercises, PNF and TENS. Two self-adhesive electrodes were applied on the anterior and posterior aspects of the shoulder joint below the acromion process (Fig. 7.16). Stimulation parameters were 200 μs pulse duration, 4 Hz frequency and intensity strong enough to produce visible muscle contractions. Mrs McC. was given a TENS unit to use at home for 1 hour at a time for as many times as was required daily to control her pain. She was told how to set up a pulley system at home for shoulder exercises and was advised to do a set programme of exercises twice a day after she applied heat to the area. She was instructed not to use TENS before the exercises as the analgesia obtained could prevent accurate assessment of her pain-free range of movement and therefore result in her 'pushing the exercises too far'.

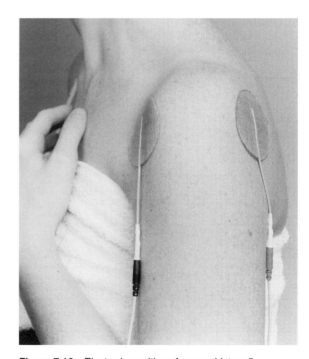

Figure 7.16 Electrode positions for case history 5.

Treatment outcome

Mrs McC. reported that the 'pulsing' effect of the TENS on her muscles gave her great pain relief and it felt 'as if the muscles were being massaged'. She used the TENS at home approximately 3–4 times a day; the last application was always just before she went to bed because this ensured a full night's sleep. By the end of the course of treatment Mrs McC. had regained full range of movement (ROM) in her left shoulder, full functional use of the left upper limb and had resumed her knitting hobby pain-free.

SUMMARY OF KEY POINTS

1. Check for any precautions prior to TENS use, then prepare the skin in order to enhance electrical conductivity.

2. Keep the first treatment short (< 30 minutes) and try conventional TENS first as it is more comfortable.

3. Choose your electrode placement sites based on the site of pain and the presence/absence of normal cutaneous sensation in the area.

4. It is desirable to use some method of pain assessment to allow monitoring of TENS treatments.

REFERENCES

Arvidsson I, Eriksson E 1986 Postoperative TENS pain relief after knee surgery: objective evaluation. Orthopedics 9(10): 1346–1351

Baldry P E 1989 Acupuncture, trigger points and musculoskeletal pain. Churchill Livingstone, Edinburgh.

Bonica J, Chadwick H S 1989 Labour pain. In: Wall P D, Melzack R (eds) Textbook of pain, 2nd edn. Churchill Livingstone, Edinburgh

Bourke D L, Smith B A C, Erickson J, Gwartz B, Lessard L 1984 TENS reduces halothane requirements during hand surgery. Anesthesiology 61(6): 769–772

Bundsen P, Ericson K 1982 Pain relief in labour by transcutaneous electrical nerve stimulation – safety aspects. Acta Obstetricia et Gynaecologica Scandinavica 61(1): 1–5

Buonocore M, Mortara A, La Rovere M T, Casale R 1992 Cardiovascular effects of TENS: heart rate variability and plethysmographic wave evaluation in a group of normal subjects. Functional Neurology 7(5): 391–394

Chapman C R, Casey K L, Dubner R, Foley K M, Gracely R H, Reading A E 1985 Pain measurement: an overview. Pain 22: 1–31

Chen A C N, Treede R D 1985 The McGill Pain Questionnaire in the assessment of phasic and tonic experimental pain: behavioral evaluation of the 'pain inhibiting pain' effect. Pain 22: 67–79

Chen D, Philip M, Philip P A, Monga T N 1990 Cardiac pacemaker inhibition by transcutaneous electrical nerve stimulation. Archives of Physical Medicine and Rehabilitation 71: 27–30

DiGregorio G J, Barbieri E J, Sterling G H, Camp J F, Prout M F 1991 Handbook of pain management, 3rd edn. Medical Surveillance, West Chester, P.A.

Dwyer C M, Chapman R S, Forsyth A 1994 Allergic contact dermatitis from TENS gel. Contact Dermatitis 30: 305

Echternach J L 1987 Pain. Clinics in physical therapy, volume 12. Churchill Livingstone, New York

Eriksson M, Schüller H, Sjölund B 1978 Hazard from transcutaneous electrical nerve stimulation in patients with pacemakers. Lancet 1: 1319

Floter T 1986 TENS treatment at home: dependence of the efficacy on frequency of use. Acupuncture and Electrotherapeutics Research International Journal 11: 153–160

Forster E L, Kramer J F, Lucy S D, Scudds R A, Novick R J 1994 Effect of TENS on pain, medications, and pulmonary function following coronary artery bypass graft surgery. Chest 106(5): 1343–1348

Fox E J, Melzack R 1976 Transcutaneous electrical stimulation and acupuncture: comparison of treatment for low-back pain. Pain 2: 141–148

Haker E, Lundeberg T 1990 Laser treatment to acupuncture points in lateral humeral epicondylalgia – a double blind study. Pain 43(2): 243–247

Harrison R F, Woods T, Shore M, Mathews G, Unwin A 1986 Pain relief in labour using transcutaneous electrical nerve stimulation (TENS): a TENS/TENS placebo controlled study in two parity groups. British Journal of Obstetrics and Gynaecology 93: 739–746

Ho A, Hui P W, Cheung J, Cheung C 1987 Effectiveness of transcutaneous electrical nerve stimulation in relieving pain following thoracotomy. Physiotherapy 73: 33–35

Jensen T S, Rasmussen P 1989 Phantom limb pain and related phenomena after amputation. In: Wall P D, Melzack R (eds) Textbook of pain, 2nd edn. Churchill Livingstone, Edinburgh

Laitinen J 1976 Acupuncture and transcutaneous electric stimulation in the treatment of chronic sacrolumbalgia and ischialgia. American Journal of Chinese Medicine 4(2): 169–175

McMichan J C, Oliver W C, Holtackers T R, Pairolero P 1985 Transcutaneous electrical nerve stimulation (TENS) for the relief of pain following thoracotomy. Anesthesia and Analgesia 64(2): 256

Mannheimer J S, Lampe G N 1984 Clinical transcutaneous electrical nerve stimulation. F A Davis, Philadelphia

Marchand S, Jinxue L, Charest J 1995 Effects of caffeine on analgesia from transcutaneous electrical nerve stimulation. New England Journal of Medicine 333(5): 325–326

Marren P, De Berker D, Powell S 1991 Methacrylate sensitivity and transcutaneous electrical nerve stimulation (TENS). Contact Dermatitis 25(3): 190–191

Melzack R 1975 The McGill Pain Questionnaire: major properties and scoring methods. Pain 1: 277–299

Melzack R, Torgerson W S 1971 On the language of pain. Anaesthesiology 34: 50–59

Melzack R, Stillwell D M, Fox E J 1977 Trigger points and acupuncture points for pain: correlations and implications. Pain 3: 3–23

Melzack R, Taenzer P, Feldman P, Kinch R 1981 Labour is still painful after childbirth. Canadian Medical Association Journal 125: 357–363

Price D D 1985 Psychological and neural mechanisms of pain. Raven Press, New York

Rasmussen M J, Hayes D L, Vlietstra R E, Thorsteinsson G 1988 Can transcutaneous electrical nerve stimulation be safely used in patients with permanent cardiac pacemakers? Mayo Clinic Proceedings 63: 443–445

Reading A E 1989 Testing pain mechanisms in persons in pain. In: Wall P D, Melzack R (eds) Textbook of pain, 2nd edn. Churchill Livingstone, Edinburgh

Swett J E, Bourassa C M 1981 Electrical stimulation of peripheral nerve. In: Patterson M M, Kesner R P (eds) Electrical stimulation research techniques. Academic Press, New York

Wall P D, Melzack R (eds) 1989 Textbook of pain, 2nd edn. Churchill Livingstone, Edinburgh

Wallenstein S L 1984 Scaling clinical pain and pain relief. In: Bromm B (ed) Pain measurements in man: neurophysiological correlates of pain. Elsevier Science, Amsterdam

Wheeler J B, Doleys D M, Harden R S, Clelland J A 1984 Conventional TENS electrode placement and pain threshold. Physical Therapy 64(5): 745

Wolf S L, Gersh M R, Rao V R 1981 Examination of electrode placements and stimulating parameters in treating chronic pain with conventional transcutaneous electrical nerve stimulation (TENS). Pain 11: 37–47

Zugerman C 1982 Dermatitis from transcutaneous electrical nerve stimulation. Journal of the American Academy of Dermatology 6(5): 936–939

CHAPTER CONTENTS

Introduction 125

Antiemetic effects 125
Postoperative – short gynaecological surgery 126
Chemotherapy 126
Postoperative – orthopaedic surgery 128
Postoperative – hysterectomy 128

Effects on circulation 128
Ischaemic tissue 128
   Reconstructive surgery – ischaemic skin flaps 128
   Chronic lower limb ischaemia 130
   Raynaud's disease/phenomenon 130
Wound healing 131
   Ulcers 131

Effects on autonomic function 132
Autonomic function in pain patients 132
Autonomic cardiovascular reflexes in healthy
  subjects 132
Hypertension 135
Coronary arterial disease 135
Coronary blood flow 136
Angina pectoris 136
Sympathetic tone/activity in healthy subjects 136

Summary of key points 137

8

Non-analgesic effects of TENS

INTRODUCTION

Although TENS devices are primarily used for pain relief, a number of non-analgesic effects have also been reported. In many cases, the accidental discovery of an interesting non-analgesic effect has inspired researchers to design further studies specifically to investigate such effects. This chapter focuses on the following three areas:

1. antiemetic effects
2. effects on circulation
3. autonomic effects.

Each of the above areas will be discussed in terms of the studies that have been reported and the postulated mechanisms of action involved. Tables 8.1–8.3 summarise the main points of the clinical studies discussed in this chapter.

ANTIEMETIC EFFECTS

As discussed in Chapter 6, one of the main disadvantages of opiate analgesics is their unwanted side-effects (nausea and vomiting are common examples). The late Professor John Dundee, of Belfast, initiated a thorough scientific investigation of the antiemetic effect of stimulation of the P6 (neiguan) acupuncture point. This acupuncture point is located 2 cun (body inches; 2 cun is the width of two thumbs; Stux & Pomeranz 1995) proximal to the distal wrist crease in line with the middle finger. Professor Dundee embarked on a series of clinical studies after observing pregnant women in China using acupressure on this point as a prophylaxis for morning sickness. Over several years, Professor Dundee and his colleagues studied the antiemetic effect of invasive and non-invasive stimulation of P6 for postoperative sickness, morning sickness and cancer chemotherapy. The application of TENS on P6 was studied in both postoperative patients and chemotherapy patients by this group (see Table 8.1).

Postoperative – short gynaecological surgery

Dundee et al (1989) reported on a series of studies carried out over a 5-year period on more than 500 female patients who had short gynaecological operations. In this series of studies, patients received routine premedication (nalbuphine 10 mg, an opiate analgesic) and anaesthesia (methohexitone-nitrous oxide-oxygen). Patients either did not receive any adjuvant therapy (controls) or received stimulation of P6 by the following methods: needle acupuncture, electroacupuncture, TENS or acupressure. Stimulation of a dummy acupuncture point was also used. All the treatments (except in one series) were applied at the time of administration of the premedication. Three different frequencies (2.5 Hz, 5 Hz and 10 Hz) of TENS were compared; stimulation was applied by a conducting stud embedded in a rubber casing. Analysis of pooled data from the various studies showed that:

- Invasive acupuncture of P6 was more effective than controls in reducing the incidence of nausea and vomiting during the first 6 postoperative hours. Stimulation of a dummy acupuncture point was not effective.
- Non-invasive methods (i.e. acupuncture and acupressure) and invasive stimulation were equally effective during the first postoperative hour, but non-invasive stimulation was less effective for the 1–6 postoperative hours.
- In the TENS applications, 10 Hz applied for 5 minutes achieved the best results.
- Stimulation of P6 before the emetic stimulus (i.e. the opiate premedication) appeared to be a critical factor in obtaining a good antiemetic effect.

Chemotherapy

The same group also investigated the antiemetic effect of P6 stimulation in chemotherapy-induced sickness (McMillan et al 1991). They compared two courses of treatments in a group of 16 cancer chemotherapy patients in a randomised crossover study. A 5-day course of chemotherapy accompanied by the antiemetic drug ondansetron was compared with a 5-day course of the same treatment with the addition of TENS; the two courses of treatment were separated by at least 3 weeks. TENS (10–15 Hz) was self-administered over P6 in the dominant forearm for 5 minutes every 2 hours when the patient was awake. The current intensity was increased to produce the sensation 'Qi', a non-anatomically distributed sensation radiating into the fingers and up the forearm. Results showed that the incidence of nausea and vomiting was less when ondansetron was combined with TENS compared to ondansetron alone.

Another paper by Dundee and colleagues (1991) described the results of pooled data from a series of studies in which TENS was compared to needle acupuncture in over 100 patients suffering from chemotherapy-induced sickness. The group of patients in this series experienced nausea and vomiting following previous courses of chemotherapy despite the use of standard antiemetics. In the studies reported, the adjuvant treatment (acupuncture or TENS) was administered before the cytotoxic drugs (i.e. chemotherapy). Patients continued to use their standard antiemetic therapy, therefore the role of complementary P6 stimulation was assessed. The key findings are summarised as follows:

- TENS was not as effective as needle acupuncture for relief of sickness; however, TENS did produce benefit in 77% of administrations.
- When acupressure was applied after needle acupuncture and TENS, it was reported that their respective antiemetic action was prolonged for 24 hours in 90% of cases.
- Best TENS results were observed with 2-hourly self-administration of 15 Hz TENS.

Table 8.1 Non-analgesic effects of TENS (antiemetic)

Reference	Condition	n	Treatment	Electrodes	Results
Dundee et al 1989 (Data pooled from several studies)	Postoperative gynae	>500	1) Control 2) Needle acupuncture 3) Electroacupuncture 4) TENS 2.5 Hz, 5 Hz and 10 Hz 5) Acupressure 6) Dummy acupuncture point	Groups 2–5 = conducting stud placed over P6. Group 6 = point outside the pericardial meridian	Less nausea with invasive acu compared with controls for 1–6 postop hours. During first hour invasive acu and non-invasive methods equally effective, after this invasive acu more effective. Of TENS frequencies, 10 Hz most effective
Dundee et al 1991 (Data pooled from several studies)	Cancer chemotherapy	>100	1) Needle acupuncture 2) TENS 10 Hz, 15 Hz and 20 Hz. Duration = 2-hourly	Conducting stud placed over P6 or cathode over P6 point and anode over Hegu point	Needle acupuncture more effective for decreasing sickness. Acupressure increased antiemetic effect of both TENS and needle acupuncture for 24 hours in 90% of cases. For TENS – 15 Hz, 2-hourly with 'Qi' was most effective
McMillan et al 1991	Cancer chemotherapy	16	1) Ondansetron 2) Ondansetron and TENS 10–15 Hz Qi elicited. Duration = 5 min every 2 hours when awake	Cathode over P6 point. Anode over Hegu point	Less nausea and vomiting with Ondansetron and TENS treatment
Fassoulaki et al 1993	Postoperative hysterectomy	106 (–3)	1) TENS 10 Hz, int just below pain 2) Placebo TENS. Duration = before anaesthesia until 6 hours postoperatively	P6 and dorsal surface of arm	Sig lower incidence in vomiting in TENS group for 6 hours postoperatively
McMillan 1994	Postoperative orthopaedic	230	1) TENS ? frequency, perceivable tingling 2) Placebo TENS 3) Subthreshold TENS. Duration of 1–3 = 5 min pre-op, then every 2 hours when awake for first 24 hours 4) Control	P6	Sig difference between groups for nausea/vomiting scores in female patients only. TENS produced best effect

Abbreviations:
Acu = acupuncture; **Int** = intensity; **Sig** = significant.
Note: the number in brackets in the 'n' column indicates the number of patients who did not complete the study.

Postoperative – orthopaedic surgery

McMillan (1994) investigated the antiemetic effect of TENS, adjunct to standard antiemetic drugs in the management of nausea and vomiting following opiate analgesia in 230 patients who had major orthopaedic surgery. Patients were randomly allocated to control, TENS, placebo TENS or subthreshold TENS groups. TENS was applied to the P6 point for 5 minutes before surgery, immediately postoperatively and then every 2 hours when the patient was awake until they were transferred to the main orthopaedic ward (pulse frequency not detailed). The incidence of nausea and vomiting was recorded using a scoring method at five time periods in the first 24 hours postoperatively. Results showed significant differences between groups (p = 0.036) for female patients only; there was a lower incidence of these symptoms in the TENS group compared with controls at the 2nd, 3rd and 4th assessment period (p < 0.001) for female patients.

Postoperative – hysterectomy

The final study in this section evaluated the antiemetic effect of TENS in 103 women undergoing hysterectomy (Fassoulaki et al 1993). Patients were allocated to a TENS or placebo TENS group (the authors call this a control group). TENS (10 Hz) was applied to P6, 30–45 minutes before the induction of anaesthesia, and remained on until 6 hours after extubation. The incidence of vomiting was assessed at 2, 4, 6 and 8 hours postoperatively. Results showed a significantly lower incidence of vomiting in the TENS group compared with placebo TENS during the 6-hour postoperative period (p < 0.005). Interestingly, the antiemetic effect disappeared when TENS was stopped (i.e. after the sixth postoperative hour).

The precise mechanism of P6 stimulation as an antiemetic is not well understood. It has been suggested that it may be mediated by stimulation of endorphin production (Post 1993). Dundee & McMillan (1991) suggest that P6 stimulation may act on a neurotransmitter involved in the transmission of neurochemical signals which play a role in emesis. Dundee et al (1990) also suggest that a psychological element appears to be involved in some circumstances. Whatever the mechanism of action, the application of TENS over P6 appears to be a successful adjunct to a standard antiemetic regime which can be easily administered by the patient.

EFFECTS ON CIRCULATION

Studies on the effects of TENS on the circulation have mainly focused on ischaemic tissue and wound healing (see Table 8.2). The first group of studies discussed below investigated the effect of electrical stimulation on ischaemic tissue.

Ischaemic tissue

Reconstructive surgery – ischaemic skin flaps

Kjartansson & Lundeberg (1990) used a crossover study design to measure blood flow in a group of 20 patients who underwent reconstructive surgery with cutaneous or fasciocutaneous flaps. All flaps in this study showed clinical signs of deficient circulation (after reconstructive surgery, ischaemia may develop leading to necrosis). Patients received TENS (0.2 ms, 90 Hz) or placebo TENS for 1 hour and then received the other treatment after a 6–10-hour rest period (these authors use the term electrical nerve stimulation (ENS) rather than TENS). After patients had received the second treatment, they then commenced a course of TENS for 2 hours twice a day until there was a significant improvement in the clinical signs of ischaemia. The electrodes were positioned on the skin at the base of the area to be treated. A laser doppler flowmeter was used to measure blood flow in the ischaemic part of the skin flaps before, during and after each treatment.

Results showed that in the crossover trial TENS treatment resulted in a significant increase in blood flow (p < 0.001) whereas placebo TENS did not. With the course of TENS treatments, there were significant improvements (p < 0.001) for capillary refill, oedema and stasis on the third

Table 8.2 Non-analgesic effects of TENS (circulation)

Reference	Condition	n	Treatment	Electrodes	Results
Kaada 1982	Peripheral ischaemia	6	TENS bursts of 5 pulses at 2 Hz, internal frequency = 100 Hz or single 0.2 ms pulses at 2–5 Hz Int = non-painful muscle contractions Duration = 30–45 minutes	One electrode placed between 1st and 2nd metacarpals, other over ulnar edge of the hand	Increase in skin temperature and decrease in pain, neither of which were affected by naloxone
Kaada 1983	Chronic ulcers	10	TENS bursts of 5 pulses at 2 Hz, internal frequency = 100 Hz Duration = 30–45 minutes × 3/day	Positive electrode over ulnar edge of the hand, negative electrode between 1st and 2nd metacarpals	Successful treatment of patients – either wound healed completely within a few weeks or the induced initial healing permitted skin grafting
Kaada & Emru 1988	Leprous ulcers	32 (−13)	TENS trains of 5 pulses at 2 Hz, internal frequency = 100 Hz, pulse duration = 0.2 ms Duration = 30 minutes × 6 am treatments and 5 pm treatments per week	Two electrodes placed locally for foot ulcers or placed either side of stump if amputee patient	All ulcers healed within a mean of 5.2 weeks
Lundeberg et al 1988	Ischaemic skin flaps	24	1) Placebo TENS Duration = 2 hours × 2/day until improvement 2) Placebo TENS and TENS 0.4 ms, 80 Hz Int = 3x tingling threshold Duration = 2 hours each treatment, then best treatment applied for 2 hours × 2/day until improvement	Two electrodes placed at base of flap	Varying degrees of necrosis developed in 8/10 placebo TENS patients, none in active TENS patients
Asbjørnsen et al 1990	Ulcers	20 (−4)	1) TENS 3 Hz trains with 100 Hz internal frequency, duration of stimulus = 85 ms Int = non-painful muscle contractions 2) Placebo TENS Duration = 30 minutes, 2/day × 5 days/week for 6 weeks	As described by Kaada 1983	The placebo TENS group had slightly better results than the TENS group
Kjartansson & Lundeberg 1990	Ischaemic skin flaps	20	1) Placebo TENS 2) TENS 0.2 ms, 90 Hz Int = 4x perception threshold Duration = 1 hour each treatment initially then course of TENS 2 hours × 2/day until sig clinical improvement	Two electrodes placed at base of area to be treated	Sig inc in blood flow with TENS treatment, not with placebo TENS. After course of TENS, significant improvement compared to post surgery
Mulder et al 1991	Raynaud's phenomenon	8	1) TENS 2 Hz Int = visible, non-painful muscle contractions 2) TENS 2 Hz Int = easily perceived but not painful Duration of 1 and 2 = 45 minutes	1 = one electrode placed between 1st and 2nd metacarpals, other over ulnar side of right hand 2 = over the middle of the iliotibial tract on right side	Vasodilation in contralateral hand and sig inc in skin temp both hands after treatment 1 No changes in transcutaneous oxygen tension in right hand
Debreceni et al 1995	Lower extremity arterial disease	24	TENS 1–2 Hz Duration = 20 minutes daily	One electrode placed between tibia and fibula, second placed between 1st and 2nd metatarsals	Improvement in all but 4 patients. Sig inc in pain-free walking distance and in oxygen saturation level in the toes

Abbreviations: Int = intensity; **Sig** = significant; **Temp** = temperature.
Note: the number in brackets in the 'n' column indicates the number of patients who did not complete the study.

day of treatment compared with post surgery values. The authors suggested that the observed effects may be due to a segmental inhibition of sympathetic vasoconstriction and the release of vasodilatory peptides from sensory neurones.

Lundeberg et al (1988) reported similar beneficial effects of TENS (again the authors use the term ENS) in a further study on fasciocutaneous flaps in a group of 24 patients who underwent reconstructive surgery for mammary carcinoma. 19 patients who showed clinical signs of stasis were randomly allocated to a TENS treatment group (n = 9) or control group (n = 10), with the remaining 5 patients (with no signs of stasis) receiving active TENS as described below. The patients allocated to the TENS treatment group received active TENS (0.4 ms, 80 Hz) and placebo TENS in a random order for 2 hours with a 6–10-hour period in between treatments (apparently only one treatment of each was given). The mode of treatment which produced the greater increase in peripheral blood flow was then applied for 2 hours twice a day until there was an improvement in capillary refilling, oedema or stasis.

As in the previous study, electrodes were positioned on the skin at the base of the flap. The placebo TENS patients received treatment for 2 hours twice a day until there was an improvement or, if there was no damage, for 7 days. A laser doppler flowmeter was used to measure peripheral blood flow; results showed varying degrees of necrosis in eight out of the 10 patients who received placebo TENS but in none of the TENS-treated patients. In the five patients who had no signs of stasis and who were treated with TENS, only minor increases in blood flow were observed.

The authors also reported that they observed the release of a potent vasodilator, calcitonin gene related peptide (CGRP) following TENS treatment in other unreferenced work: this suggests that it has a role in the observed increase in peripheral blood flow. This study was somewhat difficult to follow in terms of the allocation of patients to groups, in particular the crossover design in the TENS group added to the confusion.

Chronic lower limb ischaemia

Debreceni et al (1995) reported beneficial use of TENS for chronic lower limb ischaemia in a group of 24 patients suffering from peripheral obstructive lower limb arterial disease. In addition to standard drug therapy, TENS (1–2 Hz) was applied via two electrodes, one positioned between the tibia and head of fibula and the second in the proximal angle between the first and second metatarsals; treatment was applied daily for 20 minutes. It is unclear over what time period the patients received treatment. The interpretation of results was also unclear; the authors state that 'results are available and estimated for periods ranging for 2 months to 1 year'. Improvement was significant in all but four patients; improvement was rated in terms of a decrease in pain, cessation of the gangrenous process of the toes and regression/complete healing of ulceration. The authors reported that, after electrical stimulation, the pain-free walking distance increased significantly ($p < 0.001$) and oxygen saturation measured in the toes also increased significantly ($p < 0.05$).

Raynaud's disease/phenomenon

Raynaud's disease/phenomenon is associated with recurrent and symmetrical ischaemic attacks, primarily affecting the hands and feet. Kaada (1982) studied the effect of TENS in four patients with Raynaud's phenomenon and two with diabetic polyneuropathy (the latter two patients complained of symptoms of cold and painful legs and feet). The author tried a variety of electrode positions and reported that good vasodilation responses were regularly obtained in all four cold limbs when electrodes were positioned over the ho-ku acupuncture point (located between the first and second metacarpal bones); therefore, in this study, one electrode was placed here and the second placed over the ulnar edge of the same hand (electrodes were applied mainly on the left hand). Stimulation consisted of 0.2 ms pulses at a frequency of 2–5 Hz for 30–45 minutes; in some experiments, trains of five pulses were delivered at 2 Hz, with an internal frequency of 100 Hz. Skin temperature of the fingers and toes and pain scores were recorded every 15 minutes. Results showed that TENS produced an increase in skin temperature in the cold limbs which lasted for periods of 4–8 hours or more, this rise was associated with pain relief. The authors relate these increases to vasodilation because 'changes in skin temperature approximately reflect corresponding alterations in cutaneous vasodilation'. Interestingly, administration of naloxone intravenously at or before the beginning of the temperature rise in response to TENS did not block or reduce the observed changes in skin temperature or pain relief. As naloxone is an opiate antagonist, this suggests that opiates do not play a role in the TENS-mediated effects.

The results of Kaada's (1982) study contrast with those reported by Mulder et al (1991). Eight patients with primary Raynaud's phenomenon were treated with TENS on 2 separate days 1 week apart. On one of these days (called the TENS day), 2 Hz TENS was applied to the right first dorsal web (cathode) and ulnar side of the same hand (anode) for a 45-minute period. On the other day (called the control day), 2 Hz TENS was applied to the middle of the iliotibial tract region on the right side for a 45-minute period. Skin temperature was measured and photoelectric plethysmography performed on the third digit of both hands and feet before, during and for 4 hours after TENS. In addition, transcutaneous oxygen tension of the third digit of the right hand was measured with a radiometer. A significantly ($p < 0.05$) higher temperature was found during the 4-hour period after TENS in the right third digit on the TENS day compared to the control day.

A significantly (p value not given) higher temperature was found for the 2–4-hour period after TENS in the left third digit compared to the control day. No differences were observed for toe temperature or for transcutaneous oxygen tension of the right hand. An increase in plethysmographic amplitude, indicative of vasodilation, was observed after TENS in the left third digit. The study therefore showed a slight increase in skin temperature of both hands and vasodilation in the hand contralateral to TENS application. The authors dismissed the results of the study,

stating that they seem to be of no clinical value to Raynaud's phenomenon. The difference in stimulation parameters used in these last two studies may have contributed to the different results. In the majority of Kaada's work, trains of stimuli were delivered at a 2 Hz frequency, whereas Mulder et al used 2 Hz stimulation (trains of pulses were not mentioned). Certainly the application of TENS for ischaemic conditions such as Raynaud's disease requires further investigation.

Wound healing

Ulcers

The next four studies examined the therapeutic benefit of TENS application for the healing of ulcers. Kaada & Emru (1988) studied 19 leprosy patients who had chronic ulcers in the soft tissues of the foot or lower leg; these ulcers had resisted treatment for several months or years. In addition to standard treatment, TENS was applied for 30 minutes during six morning treatment sessions and five afternoon treatment sessions each week. Electrodes were applied locally for foot ulcers and on each side of the stump if the patient was an amputee. Stimulation consisted of trains of pulses at a frequency of 2 Hz, each train consisting of 5 pulses with an internal frequency of 100 Hz and a duration of 0.2 ms. In all 19 patients, the ulcers healed completely, with an average healing time of 5.2 weeks. This is a remarkable result as the ulcers had persisted for a mean period of 15.8 months before the TENS treatment. The authors suggested that the effects were due to TENS induction of vasodilation via a mediator, e.g CGRP or vasoactive intestinal polypeptides (VIP). Other mechanisms proposed include inhibition of sympathetic impulses by activation of a central serotonergic system or release of brain endorphins (β endorphins are known to stimulate secretion of growth hormones).

Kaada (1983) reported a further study of 10 patients with chronic leg and sacral ulcers of various aetiology which had resisted standard treatment. TENS was applied three times daily for 30–45 minutes. Stimulation was similar to that described in the previous study; low frequency bursts were delivered at a 2 Hz frequency, with a 100 Hz internal frequency. Electrodes were positioned with the cathode between the first and second metacarpals and the anode over the ulnar edge of the same hand (this electrode placement site was based on earlier work by Kaada (1982), discussed above). This paper presents individual results for each of the 10 patients; overall, the authors reported successful healing of ulcers within a few weeks (n = 8 patients), or the induced initial healing permitted skin grafting (n = 2 patients).

In the final study in this section, Asbjørnsen et al (1990) compared the effects of active and placebo TENS (authors called the latter a control group) in a group of 16 patients who also received standard treatment for ulcers on the heel or in the sacral region. TENS was given for 30 minutes twice daily, 5 days a week for 6 weeks. Each stimulus had a duration of 85 ms and consisted of a train of pulses delivered at 3 Hz with an internal frequency of 100 Hz. Electrodes were placed in the same area as described by Kaada (1983). Intensity was increased to produce contractions of adjacent muscles without pain. Results showed that the control group had slightly better results than the treatment group in terms of area of the ulcers; the authors consider this difference to be accidental.

The work described in this section has clearly demonstrated the potential of electrical stimulation to increase peripheral circulation. The contribution of Kaada's research in this area has highlighted the role of TENS in the promotion of wound healing.

EFFECTS ON AUTONOMIC FUNCTION

Some of the studies discussed in the previous section have suggested that TENS may affect peripheral blood flow by affecting sympathetic vasoconstriction. A sample of studies which have reported the effect of TENS on other autonomic activities are reviewed in this section (see Table 8.3).

Autonomic function in pain patients

In an early study, Ebersold et al (1977) monitored autonomic function in 20 patients with intractable pain (typically back pain) and 10 healthy subjects. TENS (10–100 Hz) was applied for 15 minutes to the patients' painful region or in an anatomically similar region in control subjects (the authors use the term TCS). Several variables related to autonomic function were monitored before, during and after TENS application, including BP, heart rate, skin temperature, pupil diameter and skin impedance. Analysis of results showed only two statistically significant differences:

1. the mean skin impedance of the 20 patients was lower after TENS than before ($p < 0.02$)
2. the mean systolic and diastolic BP of the 10 patients who reported pain relief with TENS was significantly higher ($p < 0.05$) in all test phases than mean pressures of the 10 patients who did not report pain relief, with the exception of diastolic pressure during TENS.

The skin impedance changes could have arisen due to a variety of reasons and were not thought to be clinically relevant. The authors thought that the differences in BP were due to individual variation and may represent a sampling error. Therefore this study has not provided any convincing evidence of TENS effects on the autonomic nervous system.

Autonomic cardiovascular reflexes in healthy subjects

In a more recent study, Sanderson et al (1995) assessed the effect of TENS on a variety of standard tests of autonomic cardiovascular reflexes in 10 healthy females. All subjects attended on 4 consecutive days, during which they randomly received either placebo TENS or active TENS (150 Hz, 0.2 ms); each subject had 2 days of active TENS and 2 days of placebo TENS. Electrodes were positioned in the centre of the chest and on the back at roughly the same level to produce segmental stimulation (unfortunately the authors were not more specific on the exact location of

Table 8.3 Non-analgesic effects of TENS (autonomic)

Reference	Investigation	n	Treatment	Electrodes	Results
Ebersold et al 1977	Autonomic function in pain patients and controls	30	TENS 10–100 Hz Duration = 15 minutes Int = minimal muscle contraction	Electrodes placed to deliver stimulation to the painful region in patients and to anatomically similar area in control subjects	Sig lower skin impedance after TENS in patients. Sig higher BP in patients who obtained pain relief with TENS in all test phases compared to those who did not get pain relief; exception was diastolic BP during TENS
Owens et al 1979	Sympathetic tone	7	TENS 75 Hz ± 25 Hz, 100 μs Int = definite sensation, avoiding discomfort or overt muscle twitching Duration = 1 minute	Electrodes placed over the ulnar groove and ulnar aspect of wrist at the point of max arterial pulsation	Immediate increase in infrared emission distal to site of TENS which persisted for several minutes after TENS
Wong & Jette 1984	Sympathetic tone	12	1) High frequency TENS 85 Hz, 100 μs 2) Low frequency TENS 2 Hz, 250 μs 3) Burst frequency TENS interrupted 85 Hz 2 bursts/sec, 7 pulses per burst Int = muscle contraction and electrical sensation 4) Placebo TENS Duration = 25 minutes	Four acupuncture points on one upper extremity. One channel = LI4 and H7 Second channel = LI10 and P6	Sig decrease in ipsilateral skin temp for 1, 2 and 3 groups immediately post treatment, not for placebo TENS. Similar trend on contralateral side.
Casale et al 1985	Sympathetic activity	10	TENS 120 Hz Int = steady tingling sensation Duration = ?	Electrodes placed over the course of the median nerve in forearm and wrist	Sig decrease in skin temperature of palm of hand and fingertips. Sig decrease in fingertip bloodflow
Kaada et al 1990	Coronary arterial disease	16	TENS trains of 5 pulses at 2 Hz, internal frequency = 100 Hz, pulse duration = 0.2 ms Int = non-painful muscle contractions 2) Placebo TENS Duration = 20 minutes	Positive electrode over ulnar border of the hand, negative electrode between 1st and 2nd metacarpals	Sig decrease in mean femoral arterial BP and systemic vascular resistance in TENS vs placebo TENS group
Kaada et al 1991	Hypertension	46	1) TENS trains of 5 pulses at 2 Hz Internal frequency = 100 Hz Pulse duration = 0.2 ms Int = non-painful muscle contractions 2) Placebo TENS Duration 45 min = short term study and 30 min 2/day for 2 weeks = long term study	Positive electrode over ulnar border of the hand, negative electrode between 1st and 2nd metacarpals	Sig lower BP in TENS vs placebo TENS group after short and long term studies
West & Colquhoun 1993	Angina pectoris	3	TENS 70 Hz Int = below painful Duration = 1 hour, 2–3/day	Electrodes placed on the back at the level of T1–T4	Dramatic and prolonged reduction in angina for all 3 patients

Table 8.3 (contd)

Reference	Investigation	n	Treatment	Electrodes	Results
Chauhan et al 1994	Coronary blood flow in patients	65	TENS 150 Hz, 300 ms Int = below painful Duration = 5 minutes	Electrodes placed 10–30 cm apart over chest wall (at site of most intense pain in those patients who had chest pain)	Sig increase in coronary blood flow in angina patients and coronary artery disease patients. No changes in coronary arterial diameters. Sig decrease in epinephrine levels in angina patients and coronary artery disease patients
Sanderson et al 1995	Autonomic cardiovascular reflexes in healthy subjects	10	1) TENS 150 Hz, 0.2 ms Int = below painful 2) Placebo TENS	Placed in centre of chest and on the back at roughly the same level to produce segmental stimulation	Sig lower inc in diastolic BP during TENS for handgrip test. No other sig differences for heart rate or BP for any other tests of autonomic cardiovascular function

Abbreviations:
Int = intensity; **Sig** = significant.

electrodes). On each day, subjects' BP and heart rate were measured while in the following positions: supine; a tilt table was used so subjects were tilted head-up to 60°; supine with a cold stimulus applied to the face; sitting to perform the Valsalva manoeuvre; and, finally, a handgrip test in which subjects maintained 30% of their maximum grip strength for 2 minutes. The only significant finding was for the handgrip test; there was a significantly lower ($p < 0.05$) rise in diastolic BP during active TENS than during placebo TENS. The authors therefore concluded that TENS appeared to have a mild inhibitory effect on reflexes which are mediated predominantly by the sympathetic nervous system.

Hypertension

Kaada et al (1991) reported successful application of TENS in 46 patients suffering from hypertension. Patients received either active TENS ($n = 25$) or placebo TENS ($n = 21$) applied to the first dorsal web between the first and second metacarpals (negative electrode) and the ulnar border of the same hand (positive electrode) (the authors do not specify which hand). This appears to be the standard electrode placement utilised in most of Kaada's work on vasodilation; indeed, similar stimulation parameters were used to that employed by Kaada & Emru (1988) mentioned in the wound healing section (i.e. stimulation consisted of trains of pulses delivered at a frequency of 2 Hz; each train consisted of 5 pulses, each of 0.2 ms duration, with an internal frequency of 100 Hz). An initial short term study was performed in the laboratory during which BP was monitored before and after a 45-minute treatment (TENS or placebo TENS) period. Then a second long term study was performed in which patients self-administered active or placebo TENS at home for 30 minutes twice daily for 2 weeks; BP recordings were made 10–12 hours after the last home treatment. Analysis of results from the short term study showed that at the end of stimulation, systolic pressure, mean arterial pressure and diastolic pressure were significantly lower for the TENS group than for the placebo TENS group ($p < 0.01$, $p < 0.01$ and $p = 0.02$ respec-

tively). After the 2-week long term study, there were similar differences between the TENS and the placebo TENS groups for all three measures of BP ($p < 0.01$, $p = 0.01$ and $p = 0.06$ respectively).

Therefore, TENS produced a depression of BP which may be associated with vasodilation. The authors suggested an opioid–serotonergic mechanism or VIP (vasoactive intestinal polypeptide) as possible neurotransmitters involved in TENS-induced vasodilation. The positive results of this study, compared to the largely negative findings in the previous two studies, strongly indicate that more clinical research is required in this area, in particular to identify the possible clinical role of low frequency TENS for hypertension.

Coronary arterial disease

In another study, Kaada et al (1990) investigated the effect of low frequency TENS on haemodynamic and metabolic changes in the heart. 16 patients with coronary arterial disease and angina pectoris undergoing preoperative cardiac catheterisation were included in the study; in contrast to the previous study, these patients were normotensive. A range of measurements including BP, cardiac output and myocardial blood flow were made before and after the application of active ($n = 8$) or placebo TENS ($n = 8$) for 20 minutes. Stimulation parameters and electrode placement were identical to those employed in the last study (Kaada et al 1991). There were no significant changes in myocardial blood flow, myocardial oxygen consumption or in the other haemodynamic parameters studied. However, a significant lowering ($p < 0.01$) of mean femoral arterial pressure and systemic vascular resistance, measured at 15 and 30 minutes after the start of treatment, was noted in the TENS group compared with the placebo TENS group. The results of this study are in general agreement with the rest of Kaada's work, that of an increase in peripheral microcirculation resulting from sympatho-inhibition after the application of low frequency TENS. The decrease in mean femoral arterial pressure of 10 mmHg in the normotensive patients in this study should be compared with the decrease in mean arterial pressure of 6 mmHg observed in the previous study of hypertensive patients (Kaada et al 1990).

Coronary blood flow

Chauhan et al (1994) performed a very detailed study which investigated the effect of TENS on coronary blood flow. Three groups of patients participated in the study: Group 1 patients had typical symptoms of angina (n = 34), Group 2 patients had significant coronary arterial disease (n = 15) and Group 3 were heart transplant patients (n = 16). Coronary blood flow velocity was measured at rest and after 5 minutes of TENS during cardiac catherisation. Electrodes were placed 10–30 cm apart over the chest wall at the site of usual pain in Group 1 and Group 2 patients (electrodes were 20 cm apart in all but three patients) and 20 cm apart on the anterior chest wall in Group 3 patients. Stimulation parameters were quite different to those used by Kaada. A high frequency (150 Hz), long pulse duration (300 ms) current was delivered for a 5-minute period. Results showed that TENS significantly increased coronary blood flow in the chest pain groups of patients (p < 0.001) but not in the transplant group. There were no significant changes in systemic haemodynamics (e.g. heart rate, BP) in any of the three groups. Suggested mechanisms of action were local production of vasodilatory substances or a direct reduction of sympathetic activity or both. The authors suggested that the site of vascular action was the microcirculation because they observed no changes in the diameter of the large epicardial coronary artery.

Angina pectoris

Mannheimer et al (1985) summarised findings from three studies which used TENS in the management of angina pectoris (not in table). TENS (70 Hz, 0.2 ms) was applied over the painful area of the chest wall for unspecified periods. The results of these studies were a reduction in pain, an increase in working capacity and decrease in

ST-segment depressions. West & Colquhoun (1993) also reported the successful management of three cases of refractory angina pectoris treated with TENS (70 Hz). Electrodes were placed over the upper thoracic spine between T1 and T4 and treatment was given for 1 hour, two or three times daily. In all three cases, the addition of TENS to a standard treatment regimen produced a dramatic and prolonged reduction in angina.

Sympathetic tone/activity in healthy subjects

The final three studies in this section have investigated the effect of TENS on sympathetic tone/ activity in healthy subjects. Wong & Jette (1984) measured skin temperature of both index fingers in a group of 12 subjects before treatment, after a 25-minute treatment period and at the end of a 25-minute post treatment period. The four treatment groups were: high frequency TENS (85 Hz, 100 μs), low frequency TENS (2 Hz, 250 μs), burst mode TENS (85 Hz, 2 bursts of 7 pulses per second, 250 μs) and placebo TENS. Subjects received each treatment on a different day. Two pairs of electrodes were positioned over the following four acupuncture points on one upper extremity: LI4 and H7, P6 and LI10. Results showed that the three active TENS treatments produced significant (p < 0.01) decreases in ipsilateral skin temperature immediately following treatment but this was not significant 25 minutes after treatment was finished. Immediately following treatment, the three active treatments produced significant decreases in skin temperature compared to the placebo TENS but not from each other. On the contralateral side, low frequency TENS produced a significant decrease (p < 0.05) in skin temperature compared to placebo and burst frequency TENS at the 25-minute post treatment recording point. This study therefore reported an increase in sympathetic activity evidenced by a decrease in fingertip skin temperature following TENS. The results of this study are in contrast to the general reports of Kaada, i.e. a decrease in sympathetic activity evidenced by an increase in skin temperature

(Kaada 1982). One factor which may have contributed to the contrasting results is that healthy subjects were used in this study compared to patients in Kaada's study.

Casale et al (1985) investigated the effect of high frequency TENS (120 Hz) on sympathetic activity assessed by strain gauge plethysmography and computerised telethermography. 10 healthy subjects received TENS via electrodes placed at the wrist and forearm over the course of the median nerve. The authors did not provide treatment time. Results showed a significant decrease in fingertip bloodflow ($p < 0.05$) and significant decreases in skin temperature of the palm of the hand ($p < 0.0005$). Fingertip measurements taken in five subjects showed significant decrease in temperature after TENS ($p < 0.0025$). Thus these results are in agreement with those of Wong & Jette (1984). In these two studies, measurements were made on the fingertips because bloodflow through the fingertips is controlled almost entirely by sympathetic vasoconstrictor nerves.

The last study in this section used infrared thermography to measure skin-surface temperature changes after 1 minute of TENS (Owens et al 1979). Seven healthy volunteers received frequency modulated TENS pulses (75 Hz ± 25 Hz, 100 µs) via two electrodes applied over the ulnar groove and ulnar aspect of the wrist (over the point of maximum arterial pulsation). All seven subjects showed immediate increases in infrared emission distal to the site of application of TENS, i.e. indirect evidence of cutaneous vasodilation and decreased sympathetic tone; this increase persisted for several minutes after TENS.

The last three studies above in conjunction with Kaada's work (Kaada 1982), have highlighted conflicting results on the effect of TENS on skin temperature. Differences in treatment regime, use of healthy subjects or patients and different electrode placement sites may have contributed to the controversy. This area needs further research because of the obvious clinical benefits to be gained if TENS has an effect on local bloodflow and temperature.

SUMMARY OF KEY POINTS

1. Convincing evidence has been provided for the antiemetic effects of TENS applied over the P6 acupuncture point.

2. The studies conducted on the effect of TENS on wound healing have produced very encouraging results.

3. The overall effects of TENS on the autonomic nervous system remain contentious; the conflicting results of the studies reported here highlight the need for further research in this area.

REFERENCES

Asbjørnsen G, Hernaes B, Molvaer G 1990 The effect of transcutaneous electrical nerve stimulation on pressure sores in geriatric patients. Journal of Clinical and Experimental Gerontology 12(4): 209–214

Casale R, Gibellini R, Bozzi M, Bonelli S 1985 Changes in sympathetic activity during high frequency TENS. Acupuncture and Electro-Therapeutics Research International Journal 10: 169–175

Chauhan A, Mullins P A, Thuraisingham S I, Taylor G, Petch M C, Schofield P M 1994 Effect of transcutaneous electrical nerve stimulation on coronary blood flow. Circulation 89: 694–702

Debreceni L, Gyulai M, Debreceni A, Szabó K 1995 Results of transcutaneous electrical stimulation (TES) in cure of lower extremity arterial disease. Angiology 46: 613–618

Dundee J W, McMillan C 1991 Positive evidence for P6 acupuncture antiemesis. Postgraduate Medical Journal 67: 417–422

Dundee J W, Ghaly R G, Bill K M, Chestnutt W N, Fitzpatrick K T J, Lynas A G A 1989 Effect of stimulation of the P6 anti-emetic point on postoperative nausea and vomiting. British Journal of Anaesthesia 63: 612–618

Dundee J W, Ghaly R G, Yang J 1990 Scientific observations on the anti-emetic action of stimulation of the P6 acupuncture point. Acupuncture in Medicine 7: 2–5

Dundee J W, Yang J, McMillan C 1991 Non-invasive stimulation of the P6 (neiguan) anti-emetic acupuncture point in cancer chemotherapy. Journal of the Royal Society of Medicine 84: 210–212

Ebersold M J, Laws E R, Albers J W 1977 Measurements of autonomic function before, during, and after transcutaneous stimulation in patients with chronic pain and in control subjects. Mayo Clinic Proceedings 52: 228–232

Fassoulaki A, Papilas K, Sarantopoulos C, Zotou M 1993 Transcutaneous electrical nerve stimulation reduces the incidence of vomiting after hysterectomy. Anesthesia and Analgesia 76: 1012–1014

Kaada B 1982 Vasodilation induced by transcutaneous nerve stimulation in peripheral ischaemia (Raynaud's phenomenon and diabetic polyneuropathy). European Heart Journal 3: 303–314

Kaada B 1983 Promoted healing of chronic ulceration by transcutaneous nerve stimulation (TNS). VASA 12: 262–269

Kaada B, Emru M 1988 Promoted healing of leprous ulcers by transcutaneous nerve stimulation. Acupuncture and Electro-Therapeutics Research International Journal 13: 165–176

Kaada B, Vik-Mo H, Rosland G, Woie L, Opstad P K 1990 Transcutaneous nerve stimulation in patients with coronary arterial disease: haemodynamic and biochemical effects. European Heart Journal 11: 447–453

Kaada B, Flatheim E, Woie L 1991 Low-frequency transcutaneous nerve stimulation in mild/moderate hypertension. Clinical Physiology 11: 161–168

Kjartansson J, Lundeberg T 1990 Effects of electrical nerve stimulation (ENS) in ischemic tissue. Scandinavian Journal of Plastic and Reconstructive Surgery and Hand Surgery 24: 129–134

Lundeberg T, Kjartansson J, Samuelsson U 1988 Effect of electrical nerve stimulation on healing of ischaemic skin flaps. Lancet 24: 712–714

McMillan C M 1994 Transcutaneous electrical stimulation of neiguan anti-emetic acupuncture point in controlling sickness following opioid analgesia in major orthopaedic surgery. Physiotherapy 80(1): 5–9

McMillan C, Dundee J W, Abram W P 1991 Enhancement of the anti-emetic action of ondansetron by transcutaneous electrical stimulation of the P6 anti-emetic point, in patients having highly emetic cytotoxic drugs. British Journal of Cancer 64: 971–972

Mannheimer C, Carlsson C-A, Vedin A, Wilhelmsson C 1985 Transcutaneous electrical nerve stimulation (TENS) in angina pectoris. International Journal of Cardiology 7: 91–95

Mulder P, Dompeling E C, van Slochteren-van der Boor J C, Kuipers W D, Smit A J 1991 Transcutaneous electrical nerve stimulation (TENS) in Raynaud's phenomenon. Angiology 42: 414–417

Owens S, Atkinson E R, Lees D E 1979 Thermographic evidence of reduced sympathetic tone with transcutaneous nerve stimulation. Anesthesiology 50: 62–65

Post A B 1993 Relief of vection-induced motion sickness. Gastroenterology 104: 665

Sanderson J E, Tomlinson B, Lau M S W et al 1995 The effect of transcutaneous electrical nerve stimulation (TENS) on autonomic cardiovascular reflexes. Clinical Autonomic Research 5: 81–84

Stux G, Pomeranz B 1995 Basics of acupuncture, 3rd edn. Springer, Berlin

West P D, Colquhoun D M 1993 TENS in refractory angina pectoris. Medical Journal of Australia 158: 488–489

Wong R A, Jette D U 1984 Changes in sympathetic tone associated with different forms of transcutaneous electrical nerve stimulation in healthy subjects. Physical Therapy 64: 478–482

CHAPTER CONTENTS

Introduction   139

Interesting developments   139

The future   140

9

Interesting developments and the future of TENS

INTRODUCTION

Due to major advances in design technology, modern TENS units bear little resemblance to early electrical stimulation apparatus, such as the Electreat (Fig. 1.1). The development of electroanalgesia since the early 1900s has resulted in an interesting sequence of events. Contemporary medical practice utilised crude forms of electrical stimulation rather successfully for pain relief without any real depth of knowledge of the relationship between electrical currents, neurophysiology and pain relief. By the mid 1960s, a mechanism of action was proposed for electrical stimulation analgesia by Melzack & Wall (1965), along with definitive clinical evidence for *transcutaneous* analgesia provided by Shealy among others (Shealy 1974); and so the 'modern' TENS was developed.

Over the past 26 years, the primary application of TENS has been for pain management. However, as discussed in Chapter 8, several non-analgesic effects of TENS have been documented which have potential clinical applications. This chapter briefly summarises interesting developments in TENS research and applications and concludes by postulating what the future holds for this modality.

INTERESTING DEVELOPMENTS

While reviewing the studies that have been published on TENS in preparation for this book, the author has identified a number of developments which are summarised as follows:

• The use of electrical stimulation to increase tissue repair is not a new concept, but recent interest in this area has produced very positive results. The work of Kaada in particular (see Ch. 8) has made a significant contribution to the application of TENS for wound healing.

• Chapter 8 has discussed the possible effects of TENS on the autonomic nervous system. Although results to date are ambiguous, this work has enormous potential, especially if the effects of TENS on reducing hypertension are investigated further.

• Chapter 8 has also highlighted the work of the late Professor Dundee and his colleagues who reported convincing results of the antiemetic effect of TENS applied on the P6 acupuncture point. As TENS can be self-administered quite easily, it makes one wonder why it is not routinely administered as an antiemetic in all hospitals. At the time of writing, research on the antiemetic effect of TENS is being conducted by members of the Rehabilitation Sciences Research Group, University of Ulster in conjunction with the Acute Pain Team, Royal Victoria Hospital, Belfast.

• Analysis of all the clinical and experimental studies included in this text has revealed the increasing popularity and apparent effectiveness of acupuncture points as a choice of electrode placement site for TENS. Many clinicians may be reluctant to try out acupuncture points for a variety of reasons, e.g. lack of knowledge of their location, scepticism of acupuncture, etc. However, the overwhelmingly positive results from well conducted studies which have used acupuncture points for a variety of clinical conditions (see Chs 6 and 8) suggest that acupuncture points should be at least considered during the selection of an electrode placement site.

• Several of the neurophysiological studies in Chapter 5 have suggested a peripheral neurophysiological blocking effect as a mechanism of action of TENS. The author has conducted several studies to investigate this and, at the time of writing, is involved in research in this area, working within the Rehabilitation Sciences Research Group, University of Ulster. In particular, this programme of work (supported by the Wellcome Trust) is focusing on parameter-specific neurophysiological effects of TENS.

• Early work on TENS tended largely to ignore the relevance of stimulation parameters but it has been encouraging to see that the relevance of manipulation of stimulation parameters has become an important focus for more recent publications on TENS.

THE FUTURE

With the considerable improvements in electrode design that have occurred over the past 10 years, it is likely that future TENS applications will primarily involve self-adhesive electrodes. The introduction of pregelled disposable electrodes has made the application of TENS considerably easier for both clinician and patient: the ease with which they can be applied and the variety of shapes and sizes currently available would suggest that the carbon rubber and wet gel application may soon be a thing of the past, that is if the manufacturers manage to make the cost of such electrodes more competitive. Electrode manufacturers have become increasingly aware that one electrode design does not suit all patients and have therefore designed electrodes to cater for individual needs, e.g. specific electrodes are recommended for extended wear, for the active patient, for sensitive skin, etc.

Future designs of TENS units will undoubtedly bring smaller, more compact units with even more stimulation parameter choices, e.g new waveforms, output types, etc. It has been encouraging to see that already certain manufacturers have adapted their available range of stimulation parameters because of the findings of clinical studies. However, there is also a danger of stimulation parameter 'saturation' in the future, i.e. the use of unnecessary stimulation parameters purely to make a unit look more 'high-tech'.

The size and shape of TENS units will continue to be modified according to patients' needs, e.g. a relatively new obstetric TENS design by NEEN Healthcare (see Ch. 10, Fig. 10.9) has incorporated a trigger switch on the unit itself which allows the user to change between continuous and burst outputs with relative ease. This is a more compact design than the traditional hand-held boost control which is typically attached to the unit by a lead (see Ch. 7, Fig 7.11).

The studies reviewed in Chapters 5, 6 and 8 provide an accurate picture of the surprisingly scarce amount of published literature available on TENS. This text has endeavoured to stress that attention to stimulation parameters and electrode placement sites is imperative in both clinical and laboratory research. The number of studies discussed in the review chapters that omitted essential information was quite surprising and makes interpretation of results very difficult; this discrepancy will hopefully become extinct in future TENS studies.

TENS has so many advantages with few side-effects/contraindications compared with other modalities, it deserves to be researched thoroughly so that optimal treatment programmes can be developed for our patients. The potential of TENS can only be addressed properly by the completion of controlled, double-blinded clinical trials and laboratory studies. The author remains optimistic that the future will bring more research on the analgesic and non-analgesic effects of TENS.

Even if more research does produce positive results for a given application of TENS, this is no guarantee that contemporary medical practice will change. There appears to be a degree of general reluctance to change current medical practice despite confirmation of successful alternatives, especially in the case of alternatives to the pharmacological management of a condition. For example, the majority of studies on the use of TENS for postoperative pain have shown favourable results in terms of pain relief, patient self-management and decreased medication, which all point to a cost-effective method of postoperative management with patient satisfaction. Yet, how many hospitals actually use TENS for postoperative pain? A further example is the positive results which have been reported on the use of TENS for dysmenorrhoea (see Ch. 6), yet how many clinicians would recommend TENS for this condition? Evidence-based practice should be a fundamental principle for all health care professions. Ideally, changes in practice should be made relatively quickly when definitive evidence emerges of an efficacious treatment. However, this is sadly not the case and many treatments are not accepted, a traditional management approach being preferred even when it is not as effective. It is hoped that the future of TENS will involve routine application of TENS in conditions such as the examples given, where its efficacy has been established.

The questionnaire discussed in Chapter 1 has confirmed that TENS is indeed a popular modality but its use is restricted by limited knowledge of optimal treatment regimes. It is hoped that this text has answered some of the queries associated with the clinical application of TENS and will thereby encourage clinicians to try TENS for different pain conditions and also to consider the non-analgesic effects of TENS. It is only through the combined efforts of clinicians and researchers that the ultimate goal of providing an optimal regime for pain management can realistically be achieved.

REFERENCES

Melzack R, Wall P D 1965 Pain mechanisms: a new theory. Science 150: 971–979

Shealy C N 1974 Six years' experience with electrical stimulation for control of pain. Advances in Neurology 4: 775–782

CHAPTER CONTENTS

Introduction   143
TENS units   143
  Lead wires   144
Electrodes   144
Other accessories   145

Manufacturers' products   146

General advice on selecting a TENS unit   154

10

TENS systems

INTRODUCTION

The aim of this final chapter is to provide an overview of currently available TENS units, lead wires, electrodes and accessories. A description of a range of TENS units manufactured both in the USA and Europe is provided, with emphasis on special features. In compiling this chapter, the author has attempted to provide a synopsis of current commercial systems; however, the following points must be stressed:

- this chapter merely provides information on a sample of the TENS products currently available; it is in no way exhaustive in terms of the entire range of products for each manufacturer listed
- the inclusion of apparatus/electrodes by specific manufacturers in this chapter does not indicate endorsement by the author
- in general, the specifications are as provided by the manufacturer.

The chapter concludes with general advice about purchasing a TENS unit.

TENS units

A standard TENS system will usually include the TENS unit itself, battery, electrodes, gel, tape, lead wires and an instruction manual, all packaged in a pouch or box (see Fig. 10.1). The majority of TENS units are battery powered, typically by a 9 V battery (disposable alkaline or rechargeable nickel-cadmium); exceptions to this are

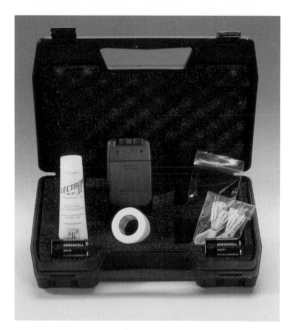

Figure 10.1   A typical TENS system (Physio-Med Services).

some multicurrent units which are powered by mains electricity.

The basic TENS unit has several features which are common to all models irrespective of individual manufacturer's preferences. The parameter controls are either analogue or digital. Analogue controls allow the adjustment of parameters by rotary dials whereas digital controls employ touch-button parameter manipulation. It is important to remember that changes in pulse amplitude, frequency or duration controls do not necessarily mean a linear change in each of these parameters; quite often, adjustments produce non-linear variations (see Chs 3 and 4, Figs 3.13, 4.2 and 4.3).

Parameter controls may be located in one area which, together with the battery compartment, is hidden beneath a removable cover. Alternatively, all the parameter controls may be visible on the exterior of the unit. The hidden compartment has the advantage of reducing the risk of the patient accidentally adjusting the controls. Dual channel units typically have independent pulse amplitude controls but only one pulse frequency and duration control to serve both channels. Some

units have a timer as an additional feature which allows the patient to set the unit to operate for up to a 1-hour period before it will automatically turn itself off.

Lead wires

Lead wires provide the important link between the base unit and the electrodes. They vary considerably in length, diameter and the number of electrodes they connect. The length of the lead wire should be long enough to allow electrodes to be positioned without a strain but short enough so that the lead wires do not get tangled; these factors are particularly important if the patient is going to be mobile while using TENS. Some lead wires connect directly to a single electrode, whereas others will divide to connect to two or four electrodes (see Fig. 10.2). It should be remembered that the greater the number of electrodes attached to a lead wire, the greater the amplitude required to deliver the required stimulus at each electrode, hence more energy will be taken from the battery.

Electrodes

Chapter 4 discussed electrode design and tissue impedance in considerable detail. The following two types of electrode design appear to be the most commonly used in TENS systems:

1. Electrodes made of carbon-loaded rubber. A layer of wet gel is applied to the electrode which is then attached to the skin by adhesive tape or, alternatively, a hydrogel pad is applied to the electrode which usually does not require tape.

2. Self-adhesive electrodes made of woven cloth (Fig. 10.3) which do not require wetting, or karaya gum which requires wetting.

Figure 10.4 illustrates a novel type of electrode which is designed for use on the back. The Lo-back® electrode (Staodyn, Inc.) is appealing as it is very easy to apply and can be cut to suit various applications.

The reader is referred to Chapter 4 for additional illustrations of electrode designs.

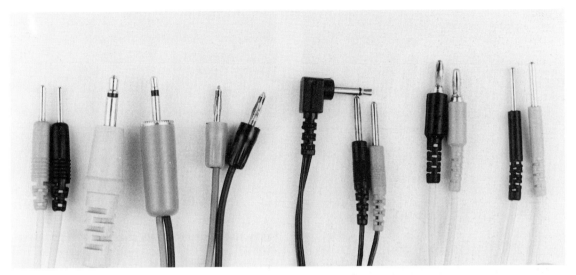

Figure 10.2 Four different sets of lead wires and their connections. Lead wires can attach directly to a single electrode as seen on the extreme right or they may bifurcate to attach to two electrodes as seen in the remaining three sets.

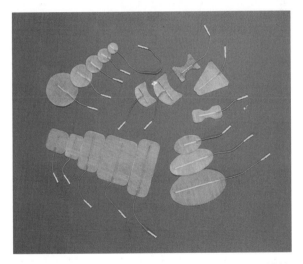

Figure 10.3 A range of self-adhesive electrodes from Nidd Valley Medical Ltd.

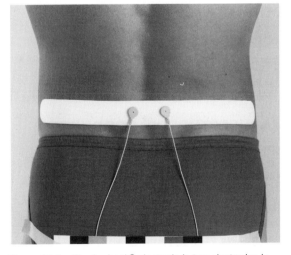

Figure 10.4 The Lo-back® electrode is two electrodes in one long strip which can be cut according to requirements (Staodyn Inc.).

Other accessories

A range of skin care products are also available as TENS accessories, these products tend to be marketed more in the USA. Figure 10.5 illustrates a sample of these products (Uni-patch Medical Supplies) which can be used for the following functions:

- Before application of TENS, wipes can be used to disinfect and cleanse the skin. In addition, skin preparation solution can be used to increase electrode adhesion and electrical conductivity.

- After TENS use, adhesive remover can be used for residual stickiness from tape or electrodes and aloe vera gel with vitamin E is available to provide relief from any unforeseen skin irritations.

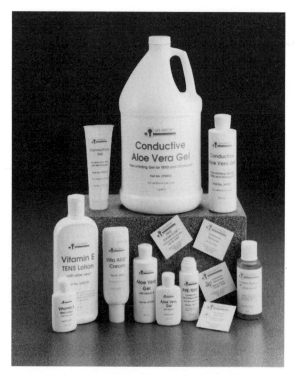

Figure 10.5   Range of skin care products (from Uni-patch Medical Supplies, P.O. Box 271, 1313 West Grant Blvd., Wabasha, MN 55981, USA).

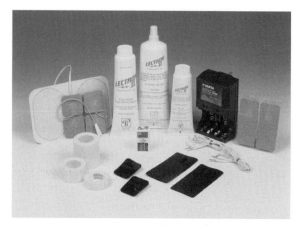

Figure 10.6   Range of TENS accessories (Physio-Med Services).

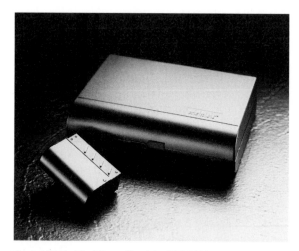

Figure 10.7   The Xenos® unit by NEEN Healthcare.

MANUFACTURERS' PRODUCTS

NEEN Healthcare

Address:

Old Pharmacy Yard
Church Street
Dereham
Norfolk NR19 1DJ
UK

   Products. The Xenos® TENS range (Fig. 10.7) consists of single or dual channel units. The single channel unit has a continuous output, fixed pulse duration (210 µs) but variable frequency controls (1–150 Hz); the dual channel unit offers adjustable pulse duration (90–300 µs) and frequency controls (1–150 Hz) and a continuous, burst or multifrequency modulation output. An important safety feature of the Xenos range is that if an electrode or lead wire becomes detached, the unit will automatically shut itself off, thereby avoiding potential uncomfortable sensa-

tions. The frequency, pulse duration and amplitude parameters are adjusted by touch controls (i.e. digital controls) rather than by movement of a dial. The dual channel unit also has a memory facility which retains the last pulse duration and frequency between uses.

   The Lifetime Microtens® range (Fig. 10.8) has three models, all of which have fixed pulse durations (200 µs) and the same frequency range (10–150 Hz). Two are single channel units with continuous or continuous/burst outputs. The third model is a dual channel unit with a continuous/burst output. All models are very compact with a control guard which protects the rotary

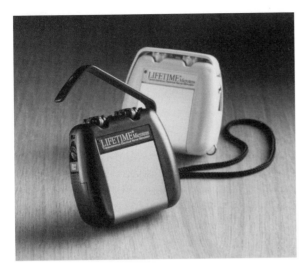

Figure 10.8 Lifetime Microtens® units by NEEN Healthcare.

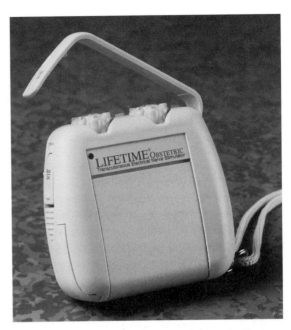

Figure 10.9 Lifetime® obstetric unit by NEEN Healthcare.

parameter controls (i.e. analogue controls) from being moved once they are set.

The Lifetime® obstetric unit (Fig. 10.9) has the same compact design as the other models in the Lifetime range. The frequency (80 Hz) and pulse duration (275 μs) parameters are both fixed. Most obstetric units have a hand-held boost control which allows the user to switch between continuous and burst outputs for the different phases of labour, i.e. during contractions / between contractions. This NEEN unit is unique in that it has incorporated a trigger switch on the side of the unit itself rather than a boost control. Because of the compact nature of this unit, it is easy to hold it in the hand and switch between the continuous and burst outputs by pressing a finger on the trigger switch.

Physio-Med Services

Address:
Hyde Park House
Cartwright Street
Newton
Hyde
Cheshire SK14 4EH
UK

Products. Physio-Med® TPN 300 model (Fig. 10.10) is a dual channel unit with variable

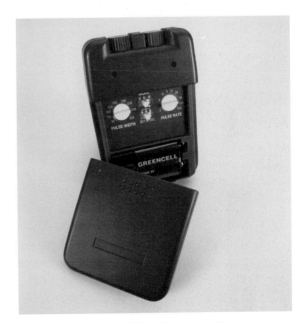

Figure 10.10 TPN 300® from Physio-Med Services.

frequency (2–150 Hz) and pulse duration (30–260 μs) parameters along with burst, normal and modulated outputs. All the parameter controls except amplitude are hidden behind a removable front panel; the amplitude is adjusted by a rotary dial on the top of the unit. As previously mentioned, this feature of a hidden parameter control area is a very good idea from a safety point of view, since it makes it impossible to accidentally adjust the hidden controls once the cover is in place.

The TPN 400® obstetric TENS (Fig. 10.11) also has a hidden parameter control area. Unlike most other obstetric units, this Physio-Med model offers an adjustable range for both frequency (2–200 Hz) and pulse duration (50–300 μs). In addition, there is a hand-held boost control with a switch at the top which allows the user to change from continuous to burst outputs. There is a 10% increase in intensity over a 3-second period when the unit is switched from burst to continuous modes which makes the change in current output more pleasant for the user.

BioMedical Life Systems, Inc.

Address:
1120 Sycamore Avenue
Suite F
Vista, California 92083
USA

Products. The Biotouch® model (Fig. 10.12) is deceptive in size in that it appears so compact that you would think it could only be a single channel unit. In fact it has two output channels on the base of the unit. The pulse duration (150 μs) and frequency (120 Hz) parameters are fixed and there is also an option of continuous or burst outputs. The output is changed by pressing the button on top of the unit. An important safety feature of this model is that the amplitude control dial is hidden behind the front cover.

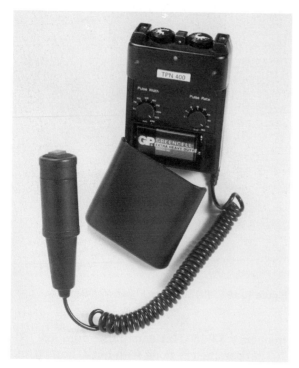

Figure 10.11   TPN 400® obstetric TENS from Physio-Med Services.

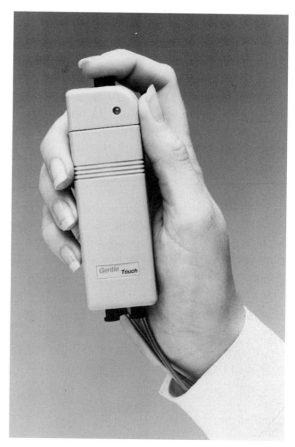

Figure 10.12   Biotouch® unit from BioMedical Life Systems, Inc.

The Systems® 2000 (Fig. 10.13) is a larger dual channel model with variable frequency (2–200 Hz) and pulse duration (10–250 µs) parameters. There is a choice of five output modes: conventional (i.e. normal), pulse rate modulation, pulse duration modulation, pulse rate and duration modulation and cycle burst. A timer control allows treatment to be set at continuous, or for 15, 30 or 60 minutes. The amplitude is adjusted by a rotary dial at the top of the unit; all other parameter controls are hidden behind the front panel.

The MFIII® unit (Fig. 10.14) is a dual channel unit which is slightly larger in size than the Systems 2000 model. This model offers a much wider range of pulse frequency than typical TENS units. There are two frequency ranges to choose from: 2–200 Hz and 8 kHz–12 kHz. Likewise there are two pulse duration ranges: 20–250 µs and 5–40 µs. This model has six modes of output: constant, burst, two pulse duration modulation and two pulse frequency modulation modes.

BMR Ltd.

Address:
Kiltartan House
Forster Street
Galway
Ireland

Product. The OmniTens® is a dual channel unit which has variable frequency (2–125 Hz) and pulse duration (80–200 µs) parameters. This sophisticated unit (Fig. 10.15) has 14 programmes, each of which offers different combinations of the range of parameters available; a switch in the battery compartment allows the clinician to set a specific programme and then the switch is moved so that the unit is ready for patient use. This important feature prevents patients altering parameters once a specific treatment programme has been set by the clinician. Another feature of this model is an LCD which can display the programme number, treatment time and amplitude. The parameters are adjusted by push button controls on the front of the unit; a desirable safety

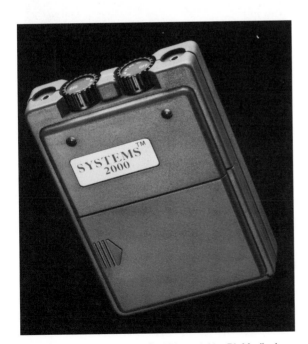

Figure 10.13 The Systems® 2000 model by BioMedical Life Systems, Inc.

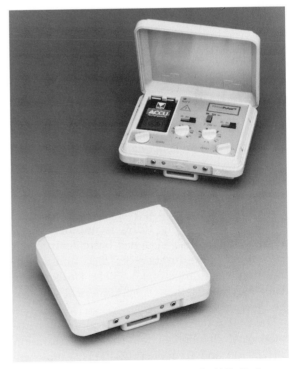

Figure 10.14 The MFIII® unit by BioMedical Life Systems, Inc.

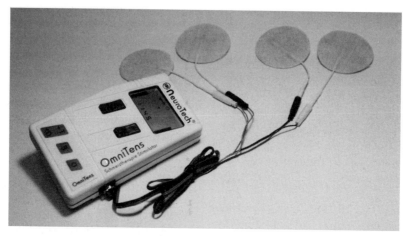

Figure 10.15   The OmniTens® unit from BMR Ltd.

feature of the OmniTens is that the amplitude control can be locked to prevent accidental movement.

Body Clock Health Care

Address:
10 Eastwood Close
South Woodford
London E18 1BX
UK

Products. The S-TENS® (Fig. 10.16) is an appealing unit in terms of the simplicity of its design. It is a single channel continuous output unit with three pulse duration settings (50, 100 and 200 µs) and a variable frequency range (1–120 Hz). Designs such as this are attractive to the patient who uses TENS at home. It should be remembered that quite often patients are put off by 'high-tech' units which appear difficult to use.

The BCT 410® (Fig. 10.17) is another single channel unit which also has basic features. It has a fixed pulse duration of 220 µs and a variable frequency range of 1.3–85 Hz. Unlike most other TENS units, there is no numerical scale for the frequency range.

The BCT 6000® (Fig. 10.18) is a more sophisticated dual channel model. The pulse duration (30–260 µs) and frequency (2–150 Hz) dials are hidden by a front panel. There are three output modes: constant, burst and amplitude modulation.

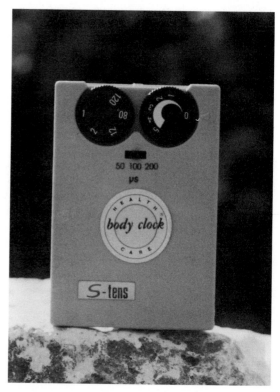

Figure 10.16   S-TENS® by Body Clock Health Care.

The V-TENS Plus® (Fig. 10.19) is rather like the BioMedical Life Systems MFIII unit in that it has two frequency ranges (2–200 Hz and 8000–12 000 Hz) and two pulse duration ranges (5–40 µs and 20–250 µs). There are four output

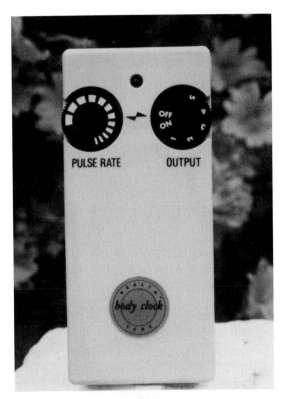

Figure 10.17   The BCT 410® unit by Body Clock Health Care.

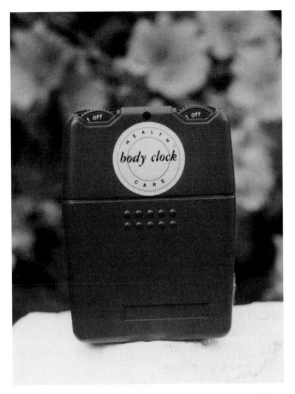

Figure 10.18   BCT 6000® model from Body Clock Health Care.

modes available: constant, burst, pulse duration modulation and frequency modulation. This unit also has a timer which allows treatment to be set at continuous or for 15, 30 or 60 minutes. All the parameter controls of this dual channel unit are hidden under the front cover, an important safety feature.

Staodyn, Inc.

Address:

1225 Florida Avenue
P.O. Box 1379
Longmount, Colorado 80502–1379
USA

Products. The Nuwave® two channel unit (Fig. 10.20) has a fixed pulse duration (60 μs) and frequency (278 Hz). There is a programmed treatment mode which involves four time periods for the current to increase to 100% intensity and then ramp off to zero intensity again. The push button controls are easy to operate and there is an indi-

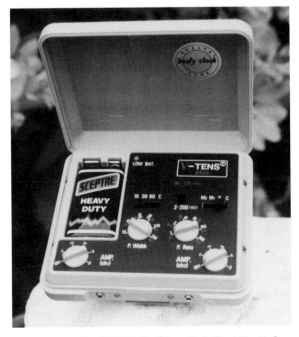

Figure 10.19   The V-TENS Plus® from Body Clock Health Care.

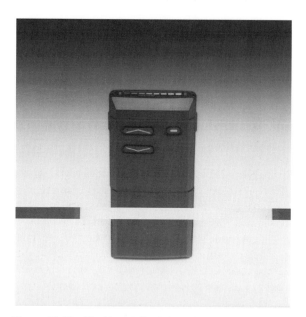

Figure 10.20   The Nuwave® unit from Staodyn, Inc.

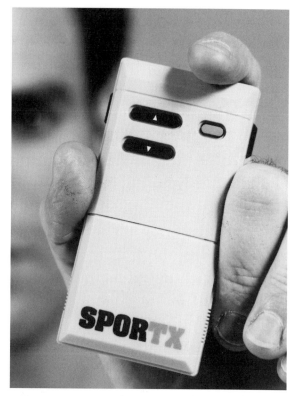

Figure 10.21   The SPORTX® model by Staodyn, Inc.

cator light which illuminates if there are battery or lead wire problems.

The SPORTX® (Fig. 10.21) is a two channel model with a difference. In this case, one channel is a typical TENS current (Nuwave® patented waveform: fixed pulse frequency 278 Hz, fixed pulse duration 60 μs) and the other is pulsed galvanic stimulation (fixed pulse frequency 222 Hz).

The Maxima II® is a dual channel TENS with variable pulse duration (50–250 μs) and pulse frequency (2–150 Hz) parameters. There are three output modes: normal, burst and modulated. A unique and desirable feature of this TENS model is a built-in test switch which will test the battery and lead wire integrity.

The Maxima III® model (Fig. 10.22) could be referred to as an upgrade version of the Maxima II model. It has also got two channels, variable frequency (2–160 Hz) and a much wider pulse duration range (50–400 μs). There are four output modes: normal, burst, modulation and strength–duration modulation; the latter mode is a recent and very unique advance in TENS units. Strength–duration modulation is based on the strength–duration curve (see Ch. 3 for details) and involves modulation of both intensity and

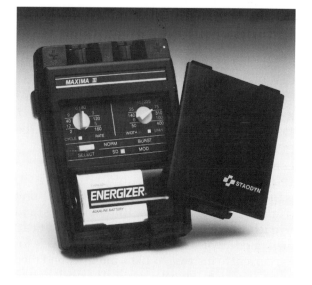

Figure 10.22   The Maxima III® model by Staodyn, Inc.

duration along the curve. The modulation is centred on the middle of the pulse duration range (i.e. 225 μs) and scans up and down the curve from this duration. Another interesting feature of this model is the 'soft turn-on' which means that if the current output is interrupted (e.g. with accidental disconnection of the lead wire), the current ramps up slowly when it resumes; this feature is important for patient comfort.

Stimtech Products, Inc.

Address:
1 Brigham Street
Marlborough, MA 01752
USA

Products. The SDM® two channel model offers a 2–200 Hz frequency range and 20–300 μs or 20–600 μs pulse duration range depending on the output mode. There are four output modes: normal, burst and two strength–duration modulation modes (SD and SSD). All parameter controls are hidden behind the front panel. A very important feature which appears on this Stimtech model is a 'use meter'; this enables the clinician to monitor the amount of time that the unit has been used by the patient. This facility will therefore allow clinicians to determine if the patient is a true non-responder or if they simply have not been using the TENS unit.

The PT1® model is another sophisticated model which also has the 'use meter' facility. This dual channel model has the same pulse duration and frequency ranges as the SDM model. The three output modes are normal, burst and amplitude/duration modulation. There is a programmable memory feature on this model which saves the parameters set by the clinician and also prevents the patient from altering them.

Tenscare Ltd.

Address:
P.O. Box 404
Kingston
Surrey KT2 7YS
UK

Products. The Unitouch® appears to be the smallest TENS unit currently available with the minute dimensions of 55 × 24 × 6 mm and only weighing 6 g. It is operated by a 3 V lithium battery. The unit is attached directly to self-adhesive electrodes, therefore there are no dangling lead wires involved. Despite its size, the Unitouch has 7 preset programmes with current amplitude adjusted by a button control.

The Tensaid III® is a dual channel unit which has rotary controls for all parameters (pulse frequency 2–200 Hz; pulse duration 50–250 μs). There are three output modes which are selected by a switch on the front of the unit: constant, burst and pulse duration modulation.

The Alpha® series consists of the Alpha plus and super models, single and dual channel units respectively. They are narrower in size than the Tensaid model and thus are easier to hold in the hand. Both have a fixed pulse duration (150 μs) and frequency (80 Hz) and constant or burst modes.

Nidd Valley Medical Ltd.

Address:
Conyngham Hall
Knaresborough
North Yorkshire HG5 9AY
UK

Products: TPT2200® is a dual channel unit with a fixed pulse duration (200 μs) and a frequency range of 10–200 Hz (Fig. 10.23). There is

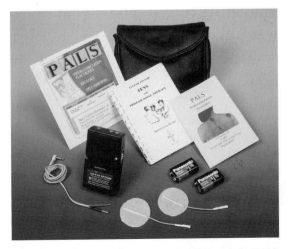

Figure 10.23 TPT2200® unit from Nidd Valley Medical Ltd.

also a higher frequency mode of 300–400 Hz. A small switch at the top of the unit allows the user to change between continuous or burst mode.

The TNS2100® model also has a fixed pulse duration (200 μs). It is preset to be switched between 100 Hz continuous or 2 Hz bursts of 100 Hz on a 20% duty cycle.

ITO Co. Ltd.

Address:
Tokyo
Japan

Product: The 120Z® dual channel unit is a robust stimulator with rotary pulse duration, frequency and intensity controls (see Fig. 10.24). There are variable frequency (2–200 Hz) and pulse duration (50–200 μs) parameters and three output modes: constant, burst and amplitude modulation. A safety lock on the pulse duration, frequency and amplitude controls prevents accidental adjustment.

GENERAL ADVICE ON SELECTING A TENS UNIT

- When selecting a unit, it should be remembered that variable frequency and pulse duration parameters, along with continuous versus burst outputs, are essential requirements in order to set the parameters required for the four modes of TENS (see Ch. 3).
- The differences between constant current and constant voltage units (discussed in Ch. 4) should be considered before purchasing a unit. All manufacturers' specifications should indicate whether their units are constant current and constant voltage.

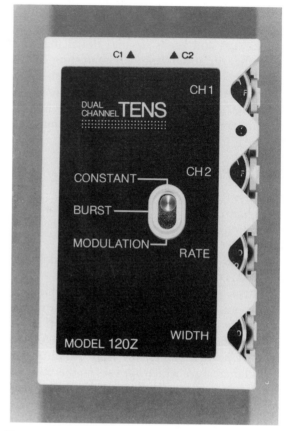

Figure 10.24 The 120Z® unit from ITO Co. Ltd.

- It is important that the design of all units should comply with safety legislation. Chapter 1 details relevant legislation for the UK, Ireland and the USA.
- As for all electrotherapy apparatus, TENS units should be calibrated regularly. Chapter 3 describes the procedure for calibration of pulse frequency and pulse duration. Chapter 3 also includes instructions on how to calculate the current output from a unit.

CHAPTER CONTENTS

Interpretation of transient responses 155
Response to an applied pulse of current 155
Current response to a pulse of voltage 157
Response to a short current pulse 157

Nonlinearity and time-dependent effects 159

Appendix I

Transient responses and nonlinearity

INTERPRETATION OF TRANSIENT RESPONSES

The response of the electrode system to sine waves of varying frequencies has been considered in Chapter 4 as this is a very useful tool in analysing the response of circuits and systems to other periodic signals. Related, but more relevant, is the response of the system (or the three-component model) to voltage and current steps or pulses. Given the effect that the electrode–skin impedance can have on the efficacy of TENS therapy, it would be advantageous to have some measure of the magnitude of impedance during TENS.

Response to an applied pulse of current

If one applies a perfect pulse of current of amplitude I_{dc} at time $t = 0$, the voltage response of the three-component model (Fig. 4.10) and, it is believed, the electrode–patient system is as shown on Figure A.1. The increase in current at $t = 0$ from zero to I_{dc} can be thought of as being equivalent to applying a very high frequency signal. This current flows unopposed through the capacitor and only 'sees' the series resistance R_S. The initial voltage response is therefore:

$$V_0 = I_{dc} R_S \qquad \text{(Equation A)}$$

One can calculate the series resistance from the voltage response by simply dividing the initial voltage V_0 by the applied DC current amplitude I_{dc}.

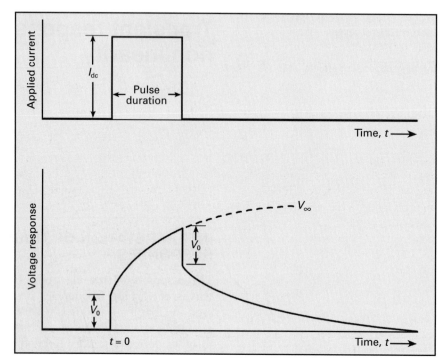

Figure A.1 Resultant voltage across the tissues in response to an applied constant current pulse of amplitude I_{dc}.

Lapsed time following the application of the step can be loosely thought of as being inversely related to the frequency of an AC signal. The magnitude of the capacitive impedance therefore increases as time passes following the application of the current step and the voltage response is observed to gradually increase from V_0. This increase in voltage with time is exponential and the rate at which the voltage increases is inversely proportional to the magnitude of the capacitance. In fact, the initial gradient is equal to I_{dc}/C_{SP}. The smaller the capacitance, the steeper the initial gradient and the more quickly the voltage response reaches its limiting value of V_∞.

(The time taken for the response to increase from the starting point of V_0 to 63% of the total increase (i.e. to $0.63\,(V_\infty - V_0)$) is called the time constant of the response, T, where $T = C_{SP}R_{SP}$. Electrode–patient impedances typically have time constants of 100 or 200 μs, see Table A.1.)

The constant voltage eventually reached by the voltage response, given sufficient time, can be thought of as the DC or low frequency re-

sponse. The current cannot flow through the capacitor and the total resistance 'seen' by the current is equal to R_S plus R_{SP}. The limit voltage, V_∞ is therefore given by:

$$V_\infty = I_{dc}\,(R_S + R_{SP}) \qquad \text{(Equation B)}$$

The voltage response will reach its limit value V_∞ in a time period of approximately five time constants. (Generally, this is considerably longer than the applied pulse duration.) In this case, the value of the parallel resistance can be calculated using Equation C.

$$R_{SP} = (V_\infty/I_{dc}) - R_S \qquad \text{(Equation C)}$$

If one subtracts V_0 from V_∞ one has:

$$V_\infty - V_0 = I_{dc}\,(R_S + R_{SP} - R_S) = I_{dc}R_{SP}$$
$$\text{(Equation D)}$$

The magnitude of the increase in voltage from V_0 is therefore proportional to the parallel resistance in the equivalent circuit model which represents the parallel resistance of the skin.

From the above, if one were to apply a sufficiently long pulse of current to the patient and if the electrode–skin interface was well represented by the proposed 'three-component' model (see Ch. 4), one could estimate the values of R_S, C_{SP} and R_{SP}.

Current response to a pulse of voltage

If a perfect pulse in voltage, V_{dc}, is applied to the electrode system or the three-component model, the current response is as shown on Figure A.2. The high frequency components associated with the rapid change at the beginning of the voltage step causes the impedance of the capacitance to be very small. Initially, therefore, the current jumps to a relatively large value I_0, where:

$$I_0 = V_{dc}/R_S \qquad \text{(Equation E)}$$

As the capacitor charges, the current then decreases exponentially with an initial slope inversely proportional to the capacitance C_{SP}. The smaller the capacitance, the more rapidly the current will decrease to its limiting value of I_∞, where:

$$I_\infty = V_{dc}/(R_S + R_{SP}) \qquad \text{(Equation F)}$$

Response to a short current pulse

The cases where a current or voltage step is applied for a sufficiently long period of time for the voltage or current response to 'settle down' and reach their 'steady state' values of V_∞ and I_∞, respectively, have been considered. If a step or pulse is applied for a length of time longer than five time constants, the conclusions stated in the previous sections will apply.

However, in order to ensure effective stimulation and minimise irritation and trauma problems, pulses of short duration are used, much shorter than the time needed to reach V_∞ or I_∞. One cannot therefore simply calculate the value of R_{SP} from the limiting values of the voltage or current responses, as before.

Many divide the measured value of the voltage at the end of a short pulse by the magnitude of

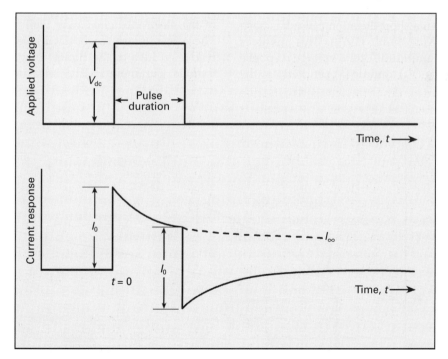

Figure A.2   Resultant current in the tissues in response to an applied constant voltage pulse of amplitude V_{dc}.

the applied current impulse and call the calculated parameter the 'instantaneous trailing edge pulse impedance' (ITEPI) (Carim 1988). It must be remembered that the magnitude of the voltage response at the end of a short impulse is a function of R_S, C_{SP} and R_{SP} and care must therefore be taken when attributing physical meaning to this calculated parameter. Nolan (1991) calculated ITEPI values for a range of electrode–skin interfaces in vivo using 200 μs, 10 mA pulses. Under these conditions, he measured ITEPI values ranging from 1000 to 7800 Ω. These values obviously very much depend on the human subject used for the experiments. The smallest ITEPI values were obtained with electrodes which were used with 'wet' gels (even in the case of carbon-loaded rubber electrodes which are intrinsically relatively resistive). The 'wet' gels presumably lead to a decrease in R_S and R_{SP} and which lead in turn to a relatively small value of voltage at the end of the applied current pulse and thus to a small ITEPI value. Karaya gel electrodes appeared to give smaller ITEPI values than many of the newer synthetic polymers.

One method of calculating the values of R_S, C_{SP} and R_{SP} from a short duration pulse has been proposed by King-Smith (1979). This involves measuring the amplitude of the voltage response at the beginning (V_0), middle (V_1) and end of the pulse (V_2). In other words, V_0 is measured at $t = 0$, V_1 at $t = T_{ph}/2$ and V_2 at $t = T_{ph}$ (Fig. A.3).

V_∞ can be calculated using the equation (Carim 1988):

$$V_\infty = I_{dc} R_{SP} + V_0 = V_0 + \frac{(V_1 - V_0)^2}{(2V_1 - V_0 - V_2)}$$

(Equation G)

One can therefore calculate the value of R_{SP}. The time constant T (where $T = R_{SP} C_{SP}$) is given by:

$$T = \frac{T_{ph}}{2 \ln \left[\dfrac{V_1 - V_0}{V_2 - V_1} \right]}$$

(Equation H)

Knowing T and R_{SP}, one can then calculate C_{SP} and compare this value with that calculated from the initial gradient (I_{dc}/C_{SP}).

Parameter values calculated using this technique for a range of electrodes attached to the skin have been kindly provided by 3M (St. Paul, Minneapolis, USA) and are reproduced with their permission on Table A.1. It must be borne in mind that these tests were carried out several years ago and that the design and performances of the electrodes cited may well have changed. These results are reproduced solely to give the reader an idea of the typical magnitudes of the various parameters. The measurements were

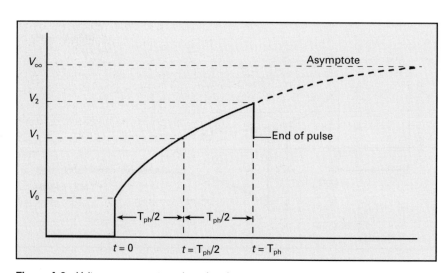

Figure A.3 Voltage response to a short duration current pulse.

carried out using 5 mA, 100 µs duration rectangular current pulses. For the given patient, under the above conditions, R_S was typically 100–500 Ω, R_{SP} was 1000–5000 Ω and C_{SP} was 0.04 to 0.1 µF. For the electrodes which have known areas (17.5 cm^2), R_{SP} was around 20 000–60 000 Ω cm^2 and C_{SP} was around 0.005–0.006 µF/cm^2. The R_{SP} values were considerably smaller than values measured using small-signal AC impedance techniques and this can be attributed to nonlinear effects (see below). The values for C_{SP} were also much smaller than those typically found for ECG 'wet' gels under small-signal conditions, the difference in this case probably being due to the TENS gels used. It should be noted that, as

the time constant of the skin's impedance is of the order of 100–250 µs, and hence equal to or more than the duration of the applied pulse, the voltage response does not have time to reach its final value (after 5 time constants). The magnitude of ITEPI, therefore, is generally much less than the sum of R_S plus R_{SP} and the values of ITEPI show little relationship, qualitative or quantitative, with the calculated values of R_{SP}.

NONLINEARITY AND TIME-DEPENDENT EFFECTS

One must bear in mind when comparing the electrical performances of various electrode systems using either small signal AC impedance techniques or a given TENS impulse amplitude, that the skin impedance is nonlinear. (The same applies to the electrode–gel interface impedance which is ignored in the present context as its contribution is relatively insignificant.) Nonlinear effects can be observed for currents above a few mA/cm^2 (Edelberg 1971) and for voltages above 2 or 3 volts (Stevens 1963). It would appear that a dramatic decrease in the skin's parallel resistance, R_{SP}, is the major cause of the observed nonlinear behaviour, with R_S unaffected and C_{SP} probably increasing slightly (Van Boxtel 1977). Large impulse amplitudes can give rise to some form of impedance 'breakdown' where the skin's impedance dramatically decreases in an 'irreversible' manner (i.e. it does not return to its linear, small-signal value upon the reduction of the applied impulse amplitude). Given sufficient time, the skin should eventually heal itself. The mechanisms involved in such breakdown are the subject of much debate. The use of such large pulses to break down the impedance of the skin prior to TENS treatment has been suggested.

It has been reported that the skin's parallel resistance appears to decrease during the duration of an applied high-amplitude pulse. There also appears to be a cumulative effect and the skin impedance progressively decreases as one continues to apply an impulse of a given amplitude. The effect may be more pronounced with applied pulses of longer durations. (It is interesting to

Table A.1 Calculated equivalent circuit parameters for a range of TENS electrodes applied to a human subject (courtesy of 3M, St. Paul, Minneapolis, USA)

Electrode	ITEPI Ω	R_S Ω	R_{SP} Ω	C_{SP} µF	T µs
Medtronic conductive rubber electrodes + 3M brand TENS gel pads (3.5 cm × 5.0 cm)	920	280	1085	0.1035	112.4
Medtronic model 3797 'Neuro Ice' electrodes	1200	150	2400	0.0724	173.8
Medtronic conductive rubber electrodes + Spectra 360 gel (3.5 cm × 5.0 cm)	1300	300	3025	0.0824	249.2
Stimtech InsTENS™ electrodes	1510	200	3990	0.0630	251.1
3M brand TENS self-adhering electrodes #6220	1610	280	2015	0.0460	87.1
3M experimental reusable, self-adhering electrodes #27	1620	400	1850	0.0502	93.1
Stimtech Dermaform™ self-adhering, disposable, TENS electrodes	1920	500	2665	0.0461	109.0

note that those who seek to electrically detect acupuncture points may in effect be creating the low impedance points they seek, in their desired locations, simply by pressing the probe on the skin and applying the measuring signal.)

The changes in the skin's parallel resistance with signal amplitude, with repeated pulsing and during an applied pulse, can have important consequences when stimulating with a constant voltage stimulator. As the amplitude of the voltage is gradually increased, there will be a disproportionate increase in the delivered current with potential risk of trauma to the patient. The time-dependent decreases in R_{SP} will lead to a progressive increase in current with time, again with potential risk to the patient.

REFERENCES

Carim H M 1988 Bioelectrodes. In: Webster J G (ed) Encyclopedia of medical devices and instrumentation. Wiley, New York

Edelberg R 1971 Electrical properties of the skin. In: Elden H R (ed) Biophysical properties of the skin. Wiley-Interscience, New York

King-Smith E A 1979 A standardized impedance measurement for TENS electrodes. Proceedings of the Annual Conference on Engineering in Medicine and Biology 21: 272

Nolan M F 1991 Conductive differences in electrodes used with transcutaneous electrical nerve stimulation devices. Physical Therapy 71: 746–751

Stevens W G S 1963 The current–voltage relationship in human skin. Medical Electronics and Biological Engineering 1: 389–399

Van Boxtel A 1977 Skin resistance during square-wave electrical pulses of 1 to 10 mA. Medical and Biological Engineering and Computing 15: 679–687

Index

*Page numbers in **bold** type refer to figures and tables.*

A

Achilles tendon reflex, 70
Action potential, 27–28
  all or none principle, 28
  compound, 18, 64
  initiation, 13, 29–30
  propagation, 28–29
  refractory period, 29
  saltatory conduction, 28–29
  speed of propagation, 29
Activation threshold, Group II fibres, 30–31
Acupressure, 125–126
Acupuncture, 108, 110
  chemotherapy sickness, 126
  points, 7
Acupuncture point P6 stimulation, 125, 126, 128, 140
Acupuncture-like TENS, 21, 36–37
  dysmenorrhoea, 84, 86
  low back pain, 88
  rheumatoid arthritis, 92, 95
Adenosine, 113
Adenosine triphosphate (ATP), 26, 27
Adhesive tape, 112
  allergic reaction, 104–105
Afferent fibres, 13–14
  characteristics, 30
  conduction velocity, 18
After-hyperpolarisation, 27
Alternating current, 32
American National Standard for Transcutaneous Electrical Nerve Stimulators (AAMI), 8
Amplifier, 41, 42
Analgesia
  stimulation produced, 20
Analgesic efficacy, 70–71
Angina pectoris, 136
Anodal block, 111
Anodal events, 31–32
Antiemetic effects of TENS, 5, 125–126, **127**, 128
Arthritis, clinical studies, 91–92, **93–94**
Aspirin, 69
Association cortex, 16
Autonomic function
  angina pectoris, 136
  cardiovascular reflexes, 132, 135
  coronary arterial disease, 135–136
  coronary blood flow, 136
  hypertension, 135
  sympathetic tone/activity, 136–137
  TENS effects, 132, **133–134**, 135–137
Autonomic nervous system, 5, 140
Axon, 25

B

BioMedical Life Systems models, 148–149
Biosignal monitoring, 59
Biotouch TENS model, 148
Blood pressure
  TENS effects, 132, 135
  see also Hypertension
Body charts, 114
Body Clock Health Care units, 150–151
Bradykinin, 13
Brainstem structures, 15–16
Brief intense TENS, 37
British Standards Institution, 7
Burn risk, 5, 44
Burst output TENS, 37, 78, 117, 154
  osteoarthritis, 95
  sympathetic tone/activity, 136

C

C fibre pain threshold, 74
C fibre-evoked flexion reflex, 68
Caffeine, 113
Calcitonin gene related peptide, 130, 131
Calcium ions, 26
Capacitance, 156, 157
  double layer (C_{dl}), 46, 48
  parallel plate capacitor, 46–47
  skin, 50–51
  stratum corneum (C_{SP}), 50
Capacitor, 46–47
  impedance, 53, **54**
Cardiac function, 104
Cardiovascular reflexes, autonomic, 132, 135
Carotid sinus, 104
Carpal tunnel syndrome, 121–122
Case histories, 119–123
Cathodal events, 31, **32**
Cerebral cortex, 16
Charge transfer
  mechanism, 45
  resistance (R_{CT}), 46, 47, 48
Chemotherapy, sickness, 126
Chi energy, 108
Chloride ions, 26
Cholecystectomy, 96
Circulation
  TENS effects, 128, **129**, 130, 132
  wound healing effects, 131–132
Clinical studies, 83–84
Clinical trial
  confounding variables, 88
  crossover, 84
  randomised controlled, 83–84
CNS metabolic activity, electrical stimulation effects, 67
Codetron TENS, 88, 92
Cognitive behaviour modification, 95

Cognitive dissonance theory, 20
Cognitive processes, pain experience, 22
Cold-induced pain, 77–78
Colles fracture, 120
Compound action potential, 18, 64, **64**
Conduction
  saltatory, 28–29
  velocity, 18, 29
Continuous output TENS, 117, 154
Contraindications for TENS, 103–105
Coronary arterial disease, 135–136
Coronary artery bypass graft surgery, 96, 118
Coronary blood flow, 136
Counterirritation, 19
Current, 32
  alternating, 32
  amplitude, 35–36
  capacitative flow, 57
  constant, 35–36, 154
  direct, 32, 33
  duration, 30
  flow, 57
  frequency, 33–34
  intensity, 35–36
    increase, 113
  output measurement, 39–40
  pulsed, 32
  response, 157
  TENS unit output, 37, 42, 44–45
  waveform, 33, 57
  see also Pulse; Pulse duration;
    Resistance
Current density, 54–55
  distribution, 45
  hot spots, 55, 57, 58
  interelectrode distance, 112
  tissue impedance, 112

D

DC voltage, 41–42
Delayed onset muscle soreness, 76–77
Dendrites, 25
Depolarisation, 27, 29, 31, **32**
  threshold, 30
  under cathode, 111
Dermatomes, 107, **109**
Dermis, 49
Descending pain suppression system, 20–22
Dielectric layer, skin, 50
Dielectric material, 47
Direct current, 32, 33
Dorsal column stimulation, 3, 4
Dorsal horn, 14–15, 19, 20
Dorsal root ganglia, 14
Double layer capacitance (C_{dl}), 46, 48
Driving, 113
Dynorphin, 20
Dysmenorrhoea, 141
  clinical studies, 84, **85**, 86

E

Electreat, 139
Electrical nerve stimulation, 75
  neuromuscular, 4
  percutaneous, 3
  transcutaneous, 4
Electrical pain, 78–79
Electricity, history as therapeutic
    modality, 2–4
Electroacupunture, 7
Electroanalgesia, 1
  history, 3
Electrocardiography, 104
Electrode gels, **50**, 51–52
  adhesive, 59
  allergic reaction, 104–105
  application, 111–112
  electrolyte concentration, 51–52, 57
  instantaneous trailing edge pulse
      impedance, 158
  ionic salt composition, 51
  pads, 59
  resistance, 51
  wet, 51–52, 55, 60
  see also Hydrogel; Karaya
Electrode–gel interface, 45–48
  capacitance, 46
Electrode–gel–skin interface, 41, 45
  circuit model, 53
  equivalent circuit model, **50**
Electrode–skin impedance, 53–54
Electrode–skin interface
  direct current, 57
  quality of contact, 52
Electrodes, 4–5, 45
  adhesive tape, 55, 56, 59
  arrangement, 111
  attachment, 58–59, 112
  carbon-loaded rubber, 59–60
  choice, 45
  conductive glue, 59
  conductive rubber, 55, 57, 60
  current density, 54–55
  design, 59–61, 140, 144
  disposable, 58, 140
  equivalent circuit parameters, **159**
  gel-retaining rings, 56
  materials, 48
  metal foil, 59, 61
  metallic layer coating, 55
  placement
    labour pain, 117
    painful area, 106, 107
    peripheral nerve, 107
    phantom limb pain, 118
    postoperative pain, 118
    sites, 160–108, 110–111
    skin flaps, 130
    specific points, 108, 110–111
    spinal nerve root, 107–108
  polarity, 111
  postoperative, 61
  pregelled, **61**
  reusable, 52
  self-adhesive, 60
  shape, 57–58
  size, 57–58
  snap fastener, 60–61
  suprapubic, 89
  surface area, 53
  totally-reusable, 60
Electrolyte gel, 45
Electromagnetic Compatibility
    Directive (89/336/EEC), 8
Electromagnetic disturbance, 8
Electrotherapeutic current, 32
Emesis see Antiemetic effects of TENS;
    Morning sickness
ß-Endorphin, 20
Endorphins
  P6 stimulation, 128
  release, 131
Enkephalins, 20
Epidermis, 49
Epilepsy, 105
Equilibrium potential, 27
Erbs point evoked potential, 64
Experimental pain, 70

F

Fast axoplasmic transport, repetitive
    stimulation effects, 67–68
Frequency of current, 33–34
Functional electrical stimulation, 4

G

Gate control theory of pain, 3, 18–19, 67
Glue, conductive, 59
Grey matter, 16
  see also Periaqueductal grey matter
Gynaecological surgery, postoperative
    TENS, 126, 128

H

H-reflex, 70
Hair follicles, 49
Hand surgery, TENS application, 118
High frequency TENS, 92, 95
  sympathetic tone/activity, 136
Holter monitor, 104
Home use, labour pain, 115
Home use of TENS, 112–113
Hydrogel, 52, 56, 57
  pad, 60
    application, 111–112
    disposable, 4–5
    sensitivity, 105
Hyperpolarisation, 32
  under anode, 111
Hypertension, 135, 140
Hypoalgesic efficacy, 71
Hysterectomy, postoperative TENS,
    128

I

Ibuprofen, 86
Ice pain threshold, 77, 78
Ileus, postoperative, 118
Impedance, 36, 155, 156, 157
  capacitative, 47, 50, 54
  capacitor, 47, 53, **54**
  electrode–skin, 53–54
  instantaneous trailing edge pulse,
      158, 159
  measure, 155
  nonlinearity, 159
  skin, 42, 48, 49, 53, 54
  stratum corneum, 50
Indomethacin, 96
Instantaneous trailing edge pulse
    impedance, 158, 159
Intensity of current, 35
Interelectrode distance, 112
Interpulse duration, 33
Ischaemic pain studies, 76
Ischaemic tissue
  blood flow stimulation, 128
  chronic lower limb, 130
  Raynaud's disease/phenomenon,
      130–131
  skin flaps, 128, 130
ITO Co. units, 154

K

Karaya, 57
  gel, 158
  pads, 105
Keratin, 49

L

Laboratory studies, 63–64
Labour, 4
  clinical studies of pain, 89, **90**, 91
  continuous application, 106
  TENS application, 115, 117
  see also Obstetric pain; Obstetric
    TENS
Latency
  measurement, 18
  somatosensory evoked potential, 69
Lateral spinothalamic tract, 15, 16
Leucine-enkephalin, 20
Limbic system, 16
Limit voltage, 156
Lissauer's tract, 14
Lo-back electrode, 144, **145**
Low back pain
  clinical studies, 86, **87**, 88

Low back pain (*contd*)
  electrode arrangement, 111
  TENS application, 120–121
  TENS comparison with ice massage, 89
Low frequency TENS, 92, 95
  sympathetic tone/activity, 136
Lower limb ischaemia, chronic, 130
Lumbar laminectomy, 99
Lung function
  postoperative, 95, 96, 99
  surgical incision site, 96
  TENS for postoperative pain, 118

M

McGill Pain Questionnaire, 115, **116**
Manufacturers' literature, 6
Manufacturing standards, 7
Maxima models, 152–153
Mechanical pain, 75
Median nerve
  sensory conduction velocity studies, 68
  somatosensory evoked potentials, 69
  stimulation studies, 68
Medical Devices Directive (93/42/EEC), 7–8
Membrane potential, 26
  development, 26–27
  ion concentration differences, 27
  resting, 26, 27, 31
  threshold potential, 28
Methionine-enkephalin, 20
Microneurographic techniques, 18, 70
Micropore tape, 112
Mixed nerves, 30–31
Morning sickness, 125–126
Morphine, 20
Motor points, 108, 111
Multisynaptic ascending system, 15, 16
Myelin sheath, 28–29
Myelinated nerve fibre, 14, 28, 29
Myofascial pain syndromes, 100
Myotome, 107

N

Naloxone, 131
Naproxen, 86, 95
Narcotics, postoperative pain, 118
Nernst equation, 27
Nerve
  conduction physiology, 25–29
  impulse *see* Action potential
  stimulation with TENS, 29–32
Nerve fibre, 25
  classification, 14
  conduction velocity, 29
  excitability changes, 64, 67
  Group II, 19
    characteristics, 30

conventional TENS, 36
  Group III, 14, 15, 17
    acupuncture-like TENS, 37
    characteristics, 30
    conductance, 31
    inhibition, 19
  Group IV, 14, 15, 17
    acupuncture-like TENS, 37
    characteristics, 30
    conductance, 31
    inhibition, 19
  myelinated, 14, 28, 29
  unmyelinated, 14, 28
Neural activity recording, 64
Neuromodulation of pain, 16
  cortical level intervention, 18
  peripheral level intervention, 17
  physiological blocking effect, 18
  spinal segmental level intervention, 17–18
  supraspinal level intervention, 18
Neuromuscular electrical stimulation, 4
Neurones, 13–14
  first order, 13
  second order, 15, 16
  structure, **26**
  third order, 16
  wide dynamic range, 15
Neurophysiological studies, 64, **65–66**, 67–70
  animal, 64, 67–68
  human, 68–70
Nickel (reaction to), 57
Nidd Valley Medical units, 153–154
Nociception, 11, 12
Nociceptive pathways
  ascending, **12**
  intervention levels, 16–18
Nociceptive signals, peripheral blockade, 18
Nociceptive specific neurones, 15
Nociceptive transmission, 21
Nociceptors, 13
Nodes of Ranvier, 29
Non-analgesic effects, 125
  autonomic function, 132, **133–134**, 135–137
  circulation, 128, **129**, 130–132
  antiemetic, 5, 125–126, **127**, 128
Noradrenaline, 20
Noxious stimuli, 12, 13
Nucleus raphe magnus, 16, 20, 21
Number of words chosen, 115
Nuwave model, 151–152

O

Obstetric analgesia, 115
Obstetric pain, 4, 6
  see also Labour
Obstetric TENS, 4, 7, 115, 117, 147, 148
  boost control, 117

clinical studies, 89, **90**, 91
  trigger switch, 117, 140
  see also Labour
Ohms law, 39
Omni TENS, 149–150
Ondansetron, 126
Opiates, 20
  nausea and vomiting, 128
  side effects, 125
Opioid–serotonergic mechanism in blood pressure depression, 135
Opioids
  endogenous, 20, 21–22
  placebo analgesia, 20
Orofacial pain, 100
Orthodromic conduction, 28
Orthopaedic surgery, postoperative TENS, 128
Oscillator, 41, 42
Oscilloscope, sweep duration, 38, 39
Osteoarthritis, 92, **93–94**
  TENS modes, 92, 95
Over-potential, 47, 48

P

P6 acupuncture point, 140
  stimulation, 125, 126, 128
Pacemakers, 104
Pain
  acute, 12
  assessment, 105, 113–115
  autonomic function, 132
  behaviour, 22
  chronic, 12
  control, 1
  definition, 12
  descending suppression system, 20–22
  descriptors, 115
  distribution, 114
  electrode placement on site, 106, 107
  emotional aspects, 16
  experience, **12**, 22
  experimental, 70
  first, 14
  induced, 76–77
  intractable, 132
  ischaemic, 76
  measurement, 113–115
  mechanical, 75
  neuromodulation, 16–18
  neurophysiology, 11–12
  perception, 11
  psychogenic, 22
  psychology, 22
  rating index, 115
  second, 14
  threshold with ice, 77, 78
  see also Low back pain; Postoperative pain; Thermal pain

Pain experimental studies, 70–71, **72–73**, 74–79
  classes, 71
  cold-induced, 77–78
  cutaneous, 71
  deep somatic, 71
  delayed onset muscle soreness, 76–77
  electrical, 78–79
  ischaemic pain, 76
  mechanical pain, 75
  model criteria, 79
  thermal pain, 71, 74–75
  value, 71
  visceral, 71
Papaveretum, 96, 98
Parallel plate capacitor, 46–47
Parallel resistance, 57, 156
  changes, 160
  nonlinear impedance, 159
Patient-controlled analgesia, 117
Patients
  competence, 104
  experience of TENS, 105–106
  motivation, 113
  preparation, 105
Periaqueductal grey matter, 16, 20, 21
  neurones, 21
Peripheral blockade of nociceptive signals, 18
Peripheral nerve
  electrode placement, 107
  mixed, 30
Peripheral neurophysiological blocking effect, 140
Phantom limb pain, 100
  electrode arrangement, 111
  TENS application, 118
Physio-Med TENS range, 147–148
Placebo
  effect, 19–20
  group, 84
Placebo TENS, sympathetic tone/ activity, 136
Polarisation, 47
Postoperative pain, 6, 95–96, **97–98**, 99–100, 141
  cholecystectomy, 96
  coronary artery bypass graft surgery, 96, 118
  gynaecological surgery, 126, 128
  hand surgery, 118
  knee surgery, 99
  orthopaedic surgery, 128
  pulmonary complications, 96, 99
  spinal surgery, 99
  thoracotomy, 96, 118
Postoperative TENS
  application, 117–118
    continuous, 106
  assessment, 96
Potassium ions, 26, 27
  efflux, 28
Precautions for TENS, 103–105

Pregnancy, 104
  acupressure, 125–126
  see also Labour
Present pain intensity, 115
Prostaglandins, 13, 84
Psychology of pain, 22
PT1 model, 153
Pulse
  amplitude, 30
  frequency calibration, 38–39, 154
  trains, 42
Pulse duration, 31, 33, 34–35
  calibration, 39, 154
  effective, 44
  short, 54, 57, 157, 158
  voltage response, 57
Pulsed current, 32

Q

Qi, 126
Quadriceps muscle contraction after knee surgery, 99
Questionnaires (McGill Pain), 115, **116**

R

Radial nerve
  A and C fibre response to stimulation, 70
  conduction latency, 68–69
Rating scales, 114
Raynaud's disease/phenomenon, 130–131
Refractory period, 29
  Group II fibres, 31
Resistance
  charge transfer (R_{CT}), 47, 48
  energy consumed by, 54
  gel, 51
  parallel, 57, 156, 159, 160
  skin, 7, 51
  stratum corneum (R_{SP}), 50
Resistor, 39
Reticular formation, 15–16
Rheumatoid arthritis, 92, **93–94**
  TENS modes, 92, 95
Rostral ventral medulla, 20, 21

S

S-TENS, 150
Saltatory conduction, 28–29
Schwann cells, 29
Sciatic nerve
  electrode arrangement for pain, 111
SDM model, 153
Segmental inhibition, 18–19
Self-management, 22
Sensation experience, 106
Sensitisation, 13

Sensory homunculus, 16
Sensory receptors, 13
Serotonergic system activation, 131
Serotonin, 20, 21
Shoulder region
  electrode placement, 112
  TENS application, 119–120, 122–123
Signal amplitude, 42
Silver-silver chloride electrodes, 48
Skin
  allergic reaction to adhesive tape, 56
  appendages, 51
  electrical properties, 49–53
  flaps, 128, 130
  impedance, 48, 49, 53
    capacitative, 54
    variation, 42
  local irritation, 54
  parallel capacitance (C_{SP}), 50–51
  parallel resistance (R_{SP}), 51
  preparation, 52
  resistance, 7, 51
  secretions, 48–49
  sensation, 103–104
  shearing stress, 55
  stripping, 52–53
  structure, 48–49
  vasodilation, 54
Skin care products, 145, **146**
Skin irritation
  chemical, 57
  current, 33
  mechanical, 55–56
  thermal, 57
Skin temperature
  sympathetic tone/activity, 136, 137
  after TENS application, 131
Skin–electrode contact, uniform, 112
Sodium ion channel inactivation, 29
Sodium ions, 26
  action potential, 28
  conductance, 29
Sodium–potassium pump, 26–27
Somatosensory cortex, 16
Somatosensory evoked potential, 64, 69
  site of application of TENS, 69–70
Spinal cord
  dorsal horn, 14–15, 19, 20
  dorsal root ganglia, 14
  segments, 107
Spinal nerve root, electrode placement, 107–108, 112
Spinal surgery, postoperative TENS, 99
Spinal tracts/pathways, 15
Spinothalamic tract cell activity inhibition, 67
SPORTX model, 152
Staodyn models, 151–153
Stimtech Products units, 153
Stimulation
  parameters, 32–36, 140
Stimulation-produced analgesia, 20
Stratum corneum, 49–50
  abrasion, 52

Strength–duration curve, 30, 31
Stretch reflex latency, 70
Subcutaneous layer of skin, 49
Submaximal effort tourniquet
        technique, 76
Substance P, 13, 14
    nociceptive transmission, 21
Substantia gelatinosa, 19
Suprathreshold stimulus, 30
Sweat ducts, 49
Sweat glands, 51
Sympathetic tone/activity, 136–137
Sympathetic vasoconstriction,
        segmental inhibition, 130
Systemic vascular resistance, 135

T

T cell, 19
TENS, 4
    advantages, 5
    adverse reactions, 5
    application site, 75
    auricular, 78–79
    available modes, 36–37
    clinical applications, 5–6
    disadvantages, 5
    early devices, 2–3
    information available, 2, 6
    nerve stimulation, 29–32
    optimal treatment parameters, 1–2
    ownership, 6–7
    placebo, 19–20, 84
    proximal application, 75
    sinusoidal, 67
    uses, 5–7
        limitations, 141
    see also Burst output TENS;
        Electrodes; High frequency
        TENS; Low frequency TENS;
        Obstetric TENS
TENS unit, 4–5, 41–42, 44–45
    amplitude control, 42, **43**
    battery powered, 41, 143
    boost control, 141
    burst output, 37
    calibration, 36, 37–40, **43**, 154
    constant current, 35–36, 154
    constant voltage, 35–36, 154
    continuous output, 37
    design, 140
    dual channel, 144, 146, 149, 150–152
    electrode circuit, 31
    lead wires, 144, **145**
    mains powered, 144
    modulated output, 37
    parameter controls, 144
    pulse duration, 57
    purchasing, 143–144
    selection, 154
    single channel, 146, 150
    trigger switch, 140
    use meter, 113, 153
    variable settings, 37
    see also Current; Electrodes
Tensaid model, 153
Tenscare units, 153
Thalamus, 16
Thermal pain
    experimental studies, 71, 74–75
Thermal sensitivity measurement, 75
Thermography, infrared, 137
Thoracotomy
    TENS application, 118
    TENS clinical study, 96
Threshold potential, 28
Tissue repair, 140
TNS2100 model, 154
TPT2200 model, 153–154
Training, 6
Transcutaneous electrical nerve
        stimulation see TENS
Transient responses, 155–159
Treatment
    duration, 106
    intensity, 106
    maximum period, 106
    regime, 105–106
Trigger points, 108, 110

U

Ulcers, 131–132
Unitouch model, 153
Unmyelinated nerve fibre, 14, 28, 54
Use meter, 113, 153

V

Vasoactive intestinal peptides, 131,
    135
Vasodilatation, 135
Vasodilatory peptide release, 130
Ventrobasal complex, 16
Verbal scales, 114
Vertebral column, 107–108
Vertebral spinous processes, 107–108,
    110
Visual analogue scale, 114–115
Voltage
    constant, 35–36, 154
    limit, 156
    response, 155

W

Waveform of current
    biphasic asymmetrical, 33
    charge-balanced biphasic, 57
    biphasic symmetrical, 33
Wide dynamic range neurones, 15
Wound healing, 5, 131–132, 140

X

XENOS TENS range, 146–147

Y

Yin/Yang, 108